PHARMACOLOGY

PEARLS OF WISDOM

Eric Scholar, Ph.D.

NOTE

The intent of PHARMACOLOGY Pearls of Wisdom is to serve as a study aid to improve performance on a standardized examination. It is not intended to be a source text of the knowledge base of medicine or to serve as a reference in any way for the practice of clinical medicine. Neither Boston Medical Publishing Corporation nor the editors warrant that the information in this text is complete or accurate. The reader is encouraged to verify each answer in several references. All drug use indications and dosages must be verified by the reader before administration of any compound.

Printed in U.S.A.

The editors would like to extend thanks to Terri Lair for her excellent managing and editorial support.

Art Director: Maryse Charette

This book was produced using Times and Symbols fonts and computer based graphics with Macintosh® computers

ISBN: 1-58409-034-0

DEDICATION

For my wife Jacqueline who has supported me when I have doubted myself.

Eric

EDITOR

Eric Scholar, Ph.D.
Associate Professor
Dept. Pharmacology
986260 Nebraska Medical Center
Omaha, NE 68198-6260
escholar@unmc.edu

WE APPRECIATE YOUR COMMENTS!

We appreciate your opinion and encourage you to send us any suggestions or recommendations. Please let us know if you discover any errors, or if there is any way we can make Pearls of Wisdom more helpful to you. We are also interested in recruiting new authors and editors. Please call, write, fax, or e-mail. We look forward to hearing from you.

Send comments to:

Boston Medical Publishing Corporation
4780 Linden Street, Lincoln, NE, 68516

888-MBOARDS (626-2737)
402-484-6118
Fax: 402-484-6552
E-mail: bmp@emedicine.com
www.bmppearls.com

INTRODUCTION

Congratulations! Pharmacology *Pearls of Wisdom* will help you pass pharmacology and improve your board scores. Pearl's unique format differs from all other review and test preparation texts. Let us begin, then, with a few words on purpose, format, and use.

The primary intent of *Pearls* is to serve as a rapid review of Pharmacology principles and serve as a study aid to improve performance on Pharmacology written and practical examinations. With this goal in mind, the text is written in rapid-fire, question/answer format. The student receives immediate gratification with a correct answer. Questions themselves often contain a "pearl" reinforced in association with the question/answer.

Additional hooks are often attached to the answer in various forms, including mnemonics, evoked visual imagery, repetition and humor. Additional information not requested in the question may be included in the answer. The same information is often sought in several different questions. Emphasis has been placed on evoking both trivia and key facts that are easily overlooked, are quickly forgotten, and yet somehow always seem to appear on Pharmacology exams.

Many questions have answers without explanations. This is done to enhance ease of reading and rate of learning. Explanations often occur in a later question/answer. It may happen that upon reading an answer the reader may think - "Hmm, why is that?" or, "Are you sure?" If this happens to you, GO CHECK! Truly assimilating these disparate facts into a framework of knowledge absolutely requires further reading in the surrounding concepts. Information learned, as a response to seeking an answer to a particular question is much better retained than that passively read. Take advantage of this. Use *Pearls* with your Pharmacology text handy and open, or, if you are reviewing on train, plane, or camelback, mark questions for further investigation.

Pearls risks accuracy by aggressively pruning complex concepts down to the simplest kernel. The dynamic knowledge base and clinical practice of medicine is not like that! This text is designed to maximize your score on a test. Refer to your mentors for direction on current practice.

Pearls is designed to be used, not just read. It is an interactive text. Use a 3x5 card and cover the answers; attempt all questions. A study method we strongly recommend is oral, group study, preferably over an extended meal or pitchers. The mechanics of this method are simple and no one ever appears stupid. One person holds *Pearls*, with answers covered, and reads the question. Each person, including the reader, says "Check!" when he or she has an answer in mind. After everyone has "checked" in, someone states his or her answer. If this answer is correct, on to the next one. If not, another person states his or her answer, or the answer can be read. Usually, the person who "checks" in first gets the first shot at stating the answer. If this person is being a smarty-pants answer-hog, then others can take turns. Try it--it's almost fun!

Pearls is also designed to be re-used several times to allow, dare we use the word, memorization. I suggest putting a check mark in each box provided every time a question is missed. Two boxes have been arbitrarily provided. If you fill all boxes on re-uses of *Pearls*, forget this question! You will get it wrong on the exam! Another suggestion is to place a check mark when the question is answered correctly once; skip all questions with check marks thereafter. Utilize whatever scheme of using the check boxes you prefer.

We welcome your comments, suggestions and criticism. Great effort has been made to verify these questions and answers. There will be answers we have provided that are at variance with the answer you would prefer. Most often this is attributable to the variance between original source (previously discussed). Please make us aware of any errata you find. We hope to make continuous improvements in a second edition and would greatly appreciate any input with regard to format, organization, content, presentation, or about specific questions. Please write to Eric Scholar, Ph.D. at . We look forward to hearing from you.

Study hard and good luck!

E.S.

TABLE OF CONTENTS

GENERAL PRINCIPLES OF PHARMACOLOGY

❑❑ **What is the therapeutic index of a drug?**

Therapeutic index (T.I.) $=LD_{50}/ED_{50}$ (ratio of toxic dose to therapeutic dose). The higher the T.I. the safer the drug.

❑❑ **What is a drug receptor?**

A macromolecular binding site which when occupied by a neurotransmitter or hormone (or agonist drug) modifies some important function of the cell through activation of an effector system.

❑❑ **What are the two main functions of drug receptors?**

The binding of the drug ligand and activation of an effector system.

❑❑ **What is a dose-response curve?**

A graphic representation of a quantitative response between the amount of drug given and the response of the drug.

❑❑ **What is the difference between a quantal dose-response curve and a graded dose-response curve?**

With a quantal dose-response curve you are looking at a population and the % of individuals responding, an either or event. At a given agonist concentration what % of the population meets that criteria. With a graded dose-response curve you relate doses of different drugs to the desired therapeutic effect in one individual.

❑❑ **What equation defines the dose-response curve?**

KA = [R] [A]/[AR]; [R] = concentration of free receptor; [A] = concentration of agonist.

❑❑ **How is a dose response curve plotted?**

The response or effect vs the agonist concentration.

❑❑ **What type of curve is defined by this equation?**

A hyperbolic curve.

❑❑ What is meant by the potency of a drug?

The amount of drug necessary to produce an effect. The concentration or dose of the drug required producing 50% of the drugs maximum effect.

❑❑ What is the efficacy of a drug?

The maximal response produced by a drug. Efficacy is often used to compare drugs.

❑❑ What is the EC_{50}?

The drug concentration required producing 50% of the maximum response.

❑❑ When the agonist concentration is equal to the KA the effect is what percentage of the maximum?

50%

❑❑ What is an inverse agonist?

A drug which has the opposite effect of an agonist.

❑❑ What is a partial agonist?

An agonist, which at even very high concentrations, gives less than 100% response. Partial agonists produce a lower response, at full receptor occupancy than do full agonists.

❑❑ What is a competitive inhibitor?

A drug which combines with the receptor and produces no response.

❑❑ What is a noncompetitive inhibitor?

It is also called an irreversible antagonist. It reduces the maximal effect without changing the potency.

❑❑ Define receptor up-regulation, down regulation and supersensitivity?

Up-regulation is an increase in the number or density of receptor binding sites. It may be reflected physiologically in an increased sensitivity of the tissue to a neurotransmitter. The term supersensitivity is often used to describe such an increased response to the drug. Down regulation is defined as a decrease in the number or density of receptor binding sites.

❑❑ What defines a receptor family?

The neurotransmitter or hormone.

❑❑ What are the four receptor superfamilies and give an example of each?

Ligand gated ion channels include the nicotinic acetylcholine receptors; G-protein coupled receptors include the beta-adrenergic receptors; tyrosine kinase receptors include growth factor receptors and nuclear receptors include the steroid receptors.

❑❑ Define pharmacokinetics and pharmacodynamics?

Pharmacokinetics defines the effect of the body on the drug while pharmacodynamics refers to the effect of the drug on the organism.

❑❑ The name of a drug that is the official name, that can only be applied to that one unique drug compound, is called what?

Generic name.

❑❑ What is the trade name of a drug?

A registered name given to the product by the pharmaceutical company that is manufacturing or distributing the drug and identifies a particular product containing that drug.

❑❑ What is drug absorption?

The transport of drugs from the site of administration into the blood.

❑❑ Name four different sites of drug administration?

Oral, inhalation, intranasal, dermal or skin, and parenterally or injection.

❑❑ What are the four different methods by which compounds cross biological membranes?

Bulk flow, passive diffusion, facilitated diffusion and active transport.

❑❑ What is passive diffusion?

The movement of drugs across lipid membranes driven down their concentration gradient.

❑❑ What is facilitated diffusion?

The carrier mediated transport of compounds down an electrochemical gradient. e.g. the cation transporter in the kidney.

❑❑ What is active transport?

An energy dependent movement of compounds across membranes against a electrochemical gradient that is carrier mediated. e.g.multidrug resistant transporters.

❑❑ What are the characteristics of active transport?

It requires energy, has substrate specificity, is saturable, involves movement against an electrochemical gradient and is inhibited by other compounds.

❑❑ How do drug transporters get their energy?

Through hydrolysis of ATP or coupling to the electrochemical gradient of another species such as Na^+ or H^+ in a symport or antiport mechanism.

❑❑ What is the Henderson-Hasselbach equation?

pKa -pH =Log (protonated)/(unprotonated)

❑❑ With a weak acid (pKa =3) is there more in the stomach or plasma after equilibrium?

There would be more in the plasma as it would be mostly unionized and therefore pass readily through the stomach.

❑❑ Would a weak acid be absorbed from the intestine?

Probably not as it would be in an ionized form.

❑❑ With a weak base (pKa=7) is there more of a weak base in the intestine or the plasma after equilibrium is established?

There would be more in the intestine as a result of more being in the ionized form.

❑❑ Consider the absorption of a weak base (pKa=7) from the intestine. Intestine pH= 6 and plasma pH=7. What % of a weak base is in the ionized form in the intestine under these conditions?

91%

❑❑ What does ion trapping mean?

When the ionized form of a drug accumulates in a tissue. Thus drugs that are highly ionized in a particular biological compartment will be trapped in that compartment.

❑❑ How would you describe the absorption of a compound charged at all physiological pHs such as quaternary amines?

They will not cross lipid membranes and thus will not be absorbed very well. They also will not enter the brain very well and they will cross the placenta very poorly unless transported by a transporter.

❑❑ What is meant by first pass metabolism?

The metabolism of the drug before the drug reaches the general circulation.

❑❑ Where does first pass metabolism usually occur?

In the stomach and intestine but mainly in the liver.

❏❏ Which route(s) of administration is most likely to subject a drug to a first-pass effect?

Oral and rectal administration. Drugs that are administered orally and rectally enter the portal circulation of the liver and can be biotransformed by this organ prior to reaching the systemic circulation.

❏❏ What sites of absorption have low first pass metabolism?

Sublingual, lungs and nasal mucosa.

❏❏ What types of delayed release preparations are available for drugs?

There are delayed release tablets, depot I.M. injections, transdermal patches, and various pumps.

❏❏ What are the advantages of oral administration of a drug?

It is most convenient to both the patient and the physician.

❏❏ What are the disadvantages of oral administration?

The taste and/or smell, and possible first pass metabolism. Also the time required for drug onset depends on site of absorption, tablet coating etc. and the amount of drug absorbed may be variable.

❏❏ Name four parenteral routes of administration?

IV, IM, SC and intrathecal.

❏❏ What is the advantage of IV drug administration?

The drug is injected directly into the blood stream. It is the most rapid and potent method of administration because the entire drug enters the circulation

❏❏ What are the advantages of sublingual administration of a drug?

There is a rapid onset and avoidance of first pass metabolism.

❏❏ What is meant by the intrathecal administration of a drug?

When a drug is injected into the spinal column.

❏❏ Drug distribution into different tissues depends on which factors?

The amount of blood flowing to the tissue vs the tissue mass, the ability of a drug to permeate the tissue, and the extent of ionization of the drug in different tissues.

❏❏ What is the most direct route of drug administration?

IV administration provides the most direct route.

❏❏ What factors must be considered in choosing a specific route of administration?

The physical and chemical characteristics of the drug., the speed at which the drug is absorbed and/or released, the need to bypass the gut or hepatic metabolism, the site of action of the drug and adverse effects of the drug at the site of administration.

❏❏ Which provides a more rapid absorption, IM or SC administration?

IM administration because of the high tissue blood flow and the ability of the injected solution to diffuse laterally.

❏❏ What are the advantages of transdermal patches?

They provide continuous drug administration and no first pass metabolism.

❏❏ What type of drugs can be given by inhalation?

Drugs that act directly on the bronchi and inhalation anesthetics.

❏❏ What are the advantages of rectal administration of drugs?

For drugs that cause GI irritation and for drugs given after GI surgery. Also it is advantageous during protracted vomiting and in uncooperative or unconscious patients.

❏❏ Which plasma proteins do drugs bind to?

Albumin, glycoprotein, and alpha and beta lipoprotein.

❏❏ What is the significance of drug-protein binding?

It affects the concentration of the free drug available. It also can lead to potential drug-drug interactions due to displacement of one drug bound to albumin by another drug.

❏❏ What is the blood-brain barrier and what is its pharmacological significance?

The blood-brain barrier refers to the row of capillary epithelial cells that regulates transfer of drugs to the brain. Only drugs having a high lipid-water partition coefficient will diffuse into the brain.

❏❏ What is the placental barrier?

The fetus and the mother are separated by a number of tissue layers that collectively constitute the placental barrier.

❏❏ What is the significance of the placental barrier?

Drugs must be able to diffuse across lipid barriers to enter the fetus.

❒❒ What is a placebo?

An inert compound identical in appearance with the drug being tested. It may or may not be known to the physician and/or patient.

❒❒ What is the name of the effect whereby two drugs acting on the same tissue or organ through independent receptors may result in opposite effects?

This is referred to as physiological antagonism.

❒❒ What is the meant by AUC (area under the blood concentration -time curve) and what does it measure?

It is the integral of the drug level over time from zero to infinity. It reflects absorption, distribution, metabolism, and excretion. It is the most reliable and popular method of evaluating bioavailability.

❒❒ How many doses of a drug are required for the plasma concentration of a drug to reach steady state if a drug is repeatedly administered at dosing intervals equal to its elimination half-life?

4-5

❒❒ Which plot is very useful for determining the total number of receptors and the affinity of a drug for those receptors in a tissue or membrane?

Scatchard plot.

❒❒ What is the importance of drug metabolism?

Metabolism is the major mechanism of drug elimination

❒❒ What happens to drugs when they are metabolized?

They are converted to products that are more polar than the parent compound.

❒❒ Is a drug always inactivated when metabolized?

Usually, but sometimes an active drug that is more potent is formed and sometimes it is first converted to a reactive intermediate.

❒❒ What are phase one reactions in drug metabolism?

Oxidation, reduction and hydrolysis reactions. These reactions introduce or expose a functional group on the compound.

❒❒ Where does the majority of drug metabolism take place?

In the liver.

❒❒ Name five other sites of drug metabolism?

The plasma, lung, kidney, intestinal mucosa, adrenals, skin and placenta

❒❒ What is the primary enzyme system involved in drug metabolism?

The cytochrome P450 system.

❒❒ What enzymes and cofactors are parts of the cytochrome P450 complex?

NADPH cytochrome P450 reductase, flavin mononucleotide, NADPH, cytochrome P450, molecular oxygen, and phosphatidylcholine

❒❒ Briefly describe the mechanism of action of drug metabolism by the cytochrome P450 system?

One molecule of oxygen is consumed for each molecule of substrate oxidized. One atom of oxygen is introduced into the substrate and the other is reduced to form water. The substrate binds to the oxidized ferric state of P450 to give a P450 drug complex. The complex then undergoes a one-electron reduction., the electron being derived from NADPH via cytochrome P450 reductase. Molecular oxygen then binds to give a ferrous cytochrome P450 dioxygen complex. A transfer of a second electron follows this from the reductase. Cleavage of the oxygen-oxygen bond then occurs concurrently with incorporation of an oxygen atom into a molecule of water, the transfer of a second oxygen atom to the substrate and the dissociation of the oxidized product.

❒❒ Where is the primary site of the cytochrome P450 system?

The liver endoplasmic reticulum.

❒❒ What are the major isoenzymes involved in the cytochrome P450 complex?

3A4, 2D6, 1A2, 2C9, and 2C19

❒❒ Give five examples of cytochrome P450 oxidation reactions?

Aromatic hydroxylations, aliphatic hydroxylations, epoxidations, oxidative dealkylations, N-oxidations, S-oxidations, deaminations, desulfurations and dechlorinations.

❒❒ What is meant by the term induction of drug metabolism?

Certain drugs or xenobiotics when administered chronically to animals and humans are shown to induce or increase cytochrome P450 isoenzymes.

❒❒ What is the significance of induction of drug metabolism?

It can result in an increased metabolism of drugs metabolized by the induced isozymes including the metabolism of the inducing agent.

❒❒ What is meant by inhibition of drug metabolism and what is its significance?

Some drugs or agents will inhibit cytochrome P450 isoenzymes. They thus can inhibit the metabolism of several drugs as well as their own metabolism.

❑❑ Name two types of reductive reactions that occur with drugs?

Azo reductions, nitro reductions, and carbonyl reductions.

❑❑ What happens during drug conjugation?

Conjugations are synthetic reactions whereby reactive groups on drugs or metabolites combine with a reactive compound found in the body.

❑❑ What happens to the drug after conjugation?

It becomes more inactive, more polar, larger and more easily excreted in the bile or urine.

❑❑ What enzyme catalyzes most conjugation reactions?

UDP-glucuronyltranferase

❑❑ What other types of conjugation reactions can occur besides glucuronidation?

Sulfate conjugation, N-acetylation, methylation reactions, glutathione conjugation and aminoacid conjugation.

❑❑ How does age effect drug metabolism?

There is less cytochrome P450 in the very young and elderly and there is decreased blood flow to the elderly.

❑❑ What type of nutritional factors effect drug metabolism?

Drug metabolism is impaired by protein deficiency. Fat free diets decrease drug metabolism. The rates of metabolism are impaired in certain vitamin deficiencies, and excessive intake of sucrose, glucose or fructose will impair monoxygenase activity.

❑❑ How do genetics affect drug metabolism?

Large differences exist among humans in their rates of plasma drug clearance and levels of some cytochrome P450 isozymes will vary between individuals.

❑❑ Explain what active tubular secretion and reabsorption in the kidney mean?

In addition to reabsorbing solutes and water, cells of the proximal tubule also secrete organic cations and organic anions. Many of these substances are end-products of metabolism and they circulate in the plasma. There are active transporters for either secretion or reabsorption. They transport either organic acids or organic bases.

❑❑ How are drugs transported into the bile from the liver?

There are transporters for anions, bile salts, cations, and neutral organic compounds.

❑❑ Explain what is meant by the term enterohepatic recirculation?

This term refers to drugs emptied via bile into the small intestine and then reabsorbed from the intestinal lumen into the systemic circulation.

❑❑ What advantage does enterohepatic cycling have for the body?

It can allow the body to conserve endogenous substances such as bile acids, vitamins D and B12, estrogen etc. It may be responsible for some of the long half-lives of drugs.

❑❑ How does antibiotic therapy interfere with the process of enterohepatic recirculation?

Drugs, which have been conjugated can be hydrolyzed by gut enzymes such as glucuronidase and then reabsorbed as the active drug or as a metabolite. A decrease in bacterial flora as a consequence of antibiotic therapy can decrease the amount of sulfatase and glucuronidase-containing bacteria. This could then lead to an increased rate of elimination of the drug.

❑❑ What are the consequences of liver disease on drug elimination?

There may be a decreased rate of drug metabolism and decreased amount of metabolites being excreted in the feces.

❑❑ What are the major pathways of drug excretion?

Renal, fecal, pulmonary, breast milk and skin.

❑❑ What types of drugs are excreted through the lungs?

Volatile substances that enter the body, e.g. inhalation anesthetics and alcohol.

❑❑ What types of drugs are excreted by way of the sweat and saliva?

Nonionized lipid forms of drugs and more hydrophilic compounds and drugs.

❑❑ What pharmacokinetic changes are seen in the very young?

There is decreased plasma protein, decreased renal clearance, changes in receptor populations, changes in end organ responsiveness, decreased drug metabolism and decreased body fat.

❑❑ What pharmacokinetic changes are seen in the elderly?

There is a decreased rate and extent of absorption as well as changes in drug distribution.

❑❑ Explain the differences between additive and synergistic effects of drugs?

Synergistic effects are effects that are greater than additive.

❑❑ What are the consequences of drug interactions?

They may result in alterations in absorption, alterations in distribution, alterations in metabolism and alterations in excretion.

❑❑ What is bioavailability?

The fraction of unchanged drug reaching the systemic circulation following administration by any route.

❑❑ What factors affect the bioavailability of a drug?

The same factors that affect absorption plus any first pass metabolism that may occur.

❑❑ What does the volume of distribution of a drug mean?

This is a hypothetical volume of body fluid that would be required to contain the entire drug administered so that the concentration will be the same as that found in the blood.

❑❑ What is drug clearance?

The body's ability to rid itself of a drug.

❑❑ How is clearance calculated?

Clearance equals the rate of elimination/concentration

❑❑ What is the plasma t 1/2 of a drug?

The time it takes for the plasma drug concentration to fall to half its initial value.

❑❑ What is the difference between first order and zero order rate of elimination of a drug?

With zero order elimination the rate of elimination is constant and independent of drug concentration. The t 1/2 depends on the amount of drug given and is longer when more of the drug has been administered. With first order elimination the t 1/2 is constant and the rate of elimination depends upon how much drug is present, being higher at higher plasma drug concentration. A constant fraction of the drug is being eliminated in unit time. Most drugs are eliminated with first-order kinetics.

❑❑ What is meant by the maintenance dose of a drug?

The amount of drug required to maintain a clinically effective concentration.

❑❑ How is the maintenance dose of a drug calculated?

Maintenance dose= dosing rate X dosing interval/bioavailability.

❑❑ What does loading dose of a drug mean?

This is the priming dose or initial dose used to initiate therapy so as to yield therapeutic concentrations that will result in clinical effectiveness.

❑❑ How is the loading dose calculated?

LD=Vd (Css-Ci) where Css and Ci refer to the steady state and initial concentrations.

❑❑ What is responsible for the different phases of a two-compartment model of drug elimination?

The rapid decline is caused mainly by the prompt redistribution of drug from the small central compartment. The second slope is caused predominantly by the elimination of the drug from the body.

❑❑ What is a pro-drug?

A compound that enters the body in an inactive form and is subsequently converted to the active form.

❑❑ What is a xenobiotic?

A compound that is foreign to the body.

DRUGS AFFECTING THE AUTONOMIC NERVOUS SYSTEM

❑❑ Cholinergic refers to what type of system?

A system where acetylcholine (Ach) is the transmitter.

❑❑ Adrenergic refers to what type of system?

A system where norepinephrine is the transmitter.

❑❑ What enzyme catalyzes the synthesis of acetylcholine?

Choline acetyltransferase

❑❑ Where is acetylcholine stored?

In the nerve terminals.

❑❑ Acetylcholine (Ach) is the transmitter at what sites?

At preganglionic fibers to all ganglia; postganglionic parasympathetic fibers to smooth muscle, heart and glands; postganglionic sympathetic fibers to sweat glands; motor fibers to skeletal muscle and in the CNS.

❑❑ Norepinephrine is the neurotransmitter at what sites?

In the CNS, at postganglionic sympathetic fibers to smooth muscle, heart and glands and in the adrenal medulla.

❑❑ How do autonomic drugs influence neurotransmission?

They can alter synthesis of the transmitter, modify the storage mechanism for neurotransmitters, change transmitter release, modify the inactivation mechanism of the transmitter and activate or block receptors. The latter is the most common mechanism.

❑❑ What are the steps in synaptic transmission?

Depolarization of presynaptic terminals, calcium influx and transmitter release. Combination of the transmitter with the postsynaptic receptor, receptor response, destruction or dissipation of the transmitter and repolarization of the postsynaptic membrane.

❑❑ **How is acetylcholine released from terminal vesicles?**

Upon arrival of an action potential and influx of calcium there is initiation of exocytosis.

❑❑ **How does botulinum toxin work?**

It inhibits the release of acetylcholine.

❑❑ **Of what use is botulinum toxin clinically?**

It is used for the treatment of certain ocular disorders, for cosmetic uses, and for spastic disorders due to neurologic injury.

❑❑ **What two types of cholinergic receptors are there?**

Muscarinic and nicotinic receptors.

❑❑ **Where are muscarinic receptors found?**

In smooth and cardiac muscle, the SA and AV nodes in the heart and exocrine glands.

❑❑ **What agents stimulate and block muscarinic receptors?**

Muscarine selectively stimulates these receptors and atropine selectively blocks them.

❑❑ **What is the mechanism of action of the muscarinic receptors?**

They are G protein coupled receptors.

❑❑ **Where are nicotinic receptors found?**

All autonomic ganglia and at the motor end-plate of skeletal muscle.

❑❑ **What agents stimulate and block nicotinic receptors?**

Nicotine selectively stimulates them. Trimethaphan blocks autonomic ganglia and tubocurarine blocks autonomic ganglia and motor fiber end-plates.

❑❑ **What is the mechanism of action of nicotine receptors?**

They are ligand gated ion channels.

❑❑ **How is cholinergic transmission terminated?**

Ach is hydrolyzed by cholinesterase enzymes.

❑❑ **What specific enzyme hydrolyzes cholinergic transmission?**

Acetylcholinesterase.

❑❑ **Where is acetylcholinesterase (AchE) found?**

At nerve endings and at the neuromuscular junction.

❑❑ **What is the function of plasma cholinesterase?**

It functions as a drug metabolizing enzyme hydrolyzing choline esters such as succinylcholine or acetylcholine (when injected).

❑❑ **Where does plasma cholinesterase occur?**

In glial cells, plasma and liver.

❑❑ **Where is norepinephrine synthesized?**

At sympathetic postganglionic nerve endings.

❑❑ **What is the rate determining enzyme in catecholamine synthesis?**

Tyrosine hydroxylase.

❑❑ **What enzyme catalyzes the synthesis of epinephrine from norepinephrine?**

Phenylethanolamine-N-methyltransferase.

❑❑ **What causes the release of norepinephrine (NE) from the synaptic vesicles?**

Calcium influx upon nerve stimulation causes the release of the vesicular contents by exocytosis.

❑❑ **What happens to transmitter release upon activation of alpha$_2$ presynaptic receptors?**

Receptor activation decreases transmitter release.

❑❑ **What is the mechanism of alpha and beta adrenergic receptors?**

They are G protein coupled receptors producing changes in cytosolic calcium or cytosolic cAMP.

❑❑ **How is norepinephrine action in the synapse terminated?**

Through uptake1, which is an active transport system.

❑❑ **What drugs inhibit this uptake system?**

Cocaine and imipramine

❑❑ **How is the action of circulating NE in the bloodstream terminated?**

Some by uptake2 located in vascular smooth muscle and glands but most by metabolism.

❑❑ What are the two main pathways for norepinephrine metabolism?

Monamine oxidase (MAO) and catechol-O-methyltransferase (COMT).

❑❑ Where are these two enzymes located?

MAO is mitochondrial and COMT is in the cytosol.

❑❑ What is the mechanism of action of MethylDOPA, tyramine, reserpine and cocaine and imipramine all of which affect adrenergic transmission?

MethylDOPA is a false transmitter; Tyramine releases NE into the synaptic cleft. Reserpine blocks dopamine uptake and depletes NE from the storage vesicle and cocaine and imipramine block uptake into the nerve ending.

❑❑ Why is acetylcholine such a poor drug?

It has poor lipid solubility, a short duration of action, and it is nonselective in its action.

❑❑ What are the effects on the cardiovascular system of acetylcholine injected IV?

There is vasodilation and negative chronotropic and inotropic effects on the atria.

❑❑ What is the mechanism of the vasodilation produced by IV acetylcholine?

It occurs through stimulation of muscarinic receptors on the endothelial cells, which results in release of nitric oxide.

❑❑ How does acetylcholine effect smooth muscle?

It increases the tone, amplitude of contraction, peristaltic activity and secretory activity of the stomach and GI tract.

❑❑ Describe the ocular effects of acetylcholine?

It contracts the sphincter muscle of the iris (miosis) and ciliary muscle (accommodation)

❑❑ What are the major pharmacological properties of bethanechol?

It produces increased smooth muscle contraction.

❑❑ What are the major pharmacological properties of pilocarpine?

Miosis, spasm of accommodation and a fall in intraocular pressure.

❑❑ What are the major toxicities of cholinomimetics?

Salivation, flushing of the skin, sweating, epigastric distress, abdominal cramps, belching, diarrhea, headache and difficulty in visual accommodation.

❑❑ **What are the antidotes for cholinomimetic toxicity?**

Atropine and epinephrine.

❑❑ **Why are cholinomimetics contraindicated in hyperthyroidism?**

They produce a reflex tachycardia.

❑❑ **Why are cholinomimetics contraindicated in asthma?**

They produce narrowing of the airways.

❑❑ **Why are cholinomimetics contraindicated in peptic ulcer?**

They produce increased acid secretion.

❑❑ **What therapeutic uses does acetylcholine have if any?**

It produces quick but short-lived miosis.

❑❑ **Why is bethanechol a preferred cholinergic drug?**

It has a preference for muscarinic receptors.

❑❑ **What is the therapeutic use of bethanechol?**

For clinical disorders that involve depression of smooth muscle activity without obstruction such as urinary retention.

❑❑ **What is pilocarpine?**

A naturally occurring cholinomimetic alkaloid obtained from the leaflets of South American shrubs.

❑❑ **How is pilocarpine used therapeutically?**

It is used to treat wide-angle glaucoma and dry mouth.

❑❑ **What is edrophonium?**

An anticholinesterase agent.

❑❑ **Why is edrophonium considered a reversible cholinesterase inhibitor?**

It only forms a weak hydrogen bond at the esteratic site.

❑❑ **What kind of a bond does neostigmine form with acetylcholinesterase?**

A hydrolyzable bond at the esteratic site.

❑❑ Why are the organophosphorus compounds irreversible cholinesterase inhibitors?

They form a covalent bond with the enzyme and new enzyme must be synthesized to overcome the effects.

❑❑ What is the mechanism of action of the anticholinesterase agents?

They result in decreased breakdown of acetylcholine through inhibition of acetylcholinesterase and direct stimulation of nicotinic receptors with some of the agents.

❑❑ What are the major pharmacokinetic properties for an anticholinesterase agent with a tertiary nitrogen like physostigmine?

They are well absorbed after oral administration and act primarily through AchE inhibition and can cross the blood brain barrier.

❑❑ What are the major pharmacokinetic properties for an anticholinesterase agent having a quaternary nitrogen like neostigmine?

There is poor absorption after oral administration, it will not readily cross the blood-brain barrier, and it acts both by AchE inhibition and by direct stimulation of nicotinic receptors.

❑❑ What are the adverse reactions of neostigmine?

It has both muscarinic (nausea and vomiting, diarrhea, abdominal cramps, salivation, sweating and miosis) and nicotinic (muscle cramps and weakness) effects.

❑❑ What is the antidote for the muscarinic actions of neostigmine?

Atropine.

❑❑ What are the pharmacological actions of neostigmine?

On the GI tract it enhances gastric contraction, increases gastric acid secretion and augments motor activity of the small and large bowel. It facilitates muscle contraction at the skeletal neuromuscular junction. At other sites it increases glandular secretions, increases the tone of smooth muscle fibers and lowers intraocular pressure.

❑❑ What are the therapeutic uses of neostigmine?

It is used to treat bladder atony, postoperative abdominal distention, myasthenia gravis and to antagonize the action of curariform drugs.

❑❑ What is meant by the term cholinergic crisis?

This is an effect caused by excessive doses of AchE inhibitors. Symptoms include miosis, sweating, salivation, lacrimation, a hyperactive bowel, muscle weakness and paralysis.

❑❑ What sites on cholinesterase are acted on by the cholinesterase inhibitors?

The anionic site and the esteratic site are sites of interaction.

❑❑ What determines the duration of cholinesterase inhibition?

The type of bond formed between the drug and the enzyme.

❑❑ Which cholinesterase inhibitor is used in the diagnosis of myasthenia gravis?

Edrophonium.

❑❑ What is physotigmine?

It is also called eserine. It is an alkaloid obtained from the Calabar or ordeal bean found in tropical West Africa. It is an anticholinesterase agent.

❑❑ What are the therapeutic uses of physotigmine?

It is used in the treatment of wide-angle glaucoma and for the reversal of anti-cholinergic toxicity.

❑❑ Which reversible cholinesterase inhibitors have been used in the treatment of Alzheimer's disease?

Donepezil and rivastigmine.

❑❑ Which of the organophosphate compounds is used clinically and why?

Echothiophate. It is used clinically because its quaternary nitrogen limits absorption and it has a long duration of action so that when instilled in the eye it stays around for awhile.

❑❑ How is echothiophate used clinically?

It is occasionally used to treat open angle glaucoma.

❑❑ Name some nerve gases that are potent anticholinesterase agents?

Tabun, sabin and soman.

❑❑ Name some insecticides that are anticholinesterase agents?

Parathion, malathion, diazinon, fenthion and chlorpyrifos.

❑❑ What is the toxicological significance of parathion?

It may be involved in accidental poisoning, suicide and homicide.

❑❑ What are the signs of nerve gas poisoning?

Same as for parathion and other cholinesterase inhibitors.

❑❑ What are the symptoms of parathion toxicity?

There are nicotinic signs (muscle weakness and fatigability) and muscarinic signs (salivation, GI hyperactivity, bronchoconstriction etc.) as well as CNS effects such as confusion, ataxia, slurred speech, loss of reflexes, generalized convulsions and respiratory paralysis.

❑❑ How are parathion poisoning as well as poisoning with other irreversible cholinesterases treated?

It depends on how soon after the patient is seen. The area should be decontaminated then respiration supported and then atropine and pralidoxime can be used as antidotes.

❑❑ What is pralidoxime?

A cholinesterase reactivator.

❑❑ What is the rationale for the use of pralidoxime?

It is very reactive with phosphorylated enzymes. It is causes reactivation of phosphorylated acetylcholinesterase.

❑❑ How does pyridostigmine compare to other cholinesterase inhibitors?

It has a longer duration of action than neostigmine.

❑❑ What is the therapeutic use of pyridostigmine?

It is the drug of choice for myasthenia gravis.

❑❑ What is isoflurophate used for?

Wide angle glaucoma (late stages).

❑❑ What toxic effect is associated with the use of isoflurophate?

Cataracts.

❑❑ What are the signs of mushroom poisoning due to muscarine containing mushrooms?

The usual signs of muscarine excess including nausea, vomiting, diarrhea, vasodilatation, reflex tachycardia, sweating, salivation and possible bronchoconstriction.

❑❑ How is mushroom poisoning due to muscarine containing mushrooms treated?

It is treated with atropine.

❑❑ What are the belladonna alkaloids?

A group of alkaloids isolated from plants related to deadly nightshade. They have antimuscarinic effects.

❑❑ Name the belladonna alkaloids?

Atropine and scopolamine.

❑❑ What are the sites of action of atropine?

It acts at muscarinic receptors, including those in blood vessels, sweat glands and the CNS.

❑❑ What is the mechanism of action of atropine and other belladonna alkaloids?

They antagonize the action of Ach at muscarinic cholinergic receptors. Only at large doses do they act at nicotinic cholinergic receptors.

❑❑ What is the order in which different tissues are effected by increasing doses of atropine?

Receptor blockade depends on the dose of atropine. Salivary and bronchial secretions and sweating are depressed first. Then mydriasis, cycloplegia and vagal blockade of the heart occur, then tone and motility of the GI tract and urinary bladder are affected and finally gastric secretion is partially inhibited.

❑❑ How does atropine effect the CNS?

At a low doses it causes mild vagal stimulation and at larger doses it causes restlessness, excitement, irritability and hallucinations.

❑❑ How does scopolamine affect the CNS?

There is a CNS depressant effect at low doses and stimulation at high doses.

❑❑ What are the ocular effects of atropine?

Mydriasis, cycloplegia and photophobia.

❑❑ Why does atropine cause tachycardia?

It occurs as a result of vagal blockade.

❑❑ What is the effect of atropine on the respiratory system?

It decreases bronchial secretions and relaxes bronchial smooth muscle.

❑❑ What are the GI effects of atropine?

It inhibits salivary secretions and reduces the tone and motility of the GI tract. There is also a partial reduction of gastric secretion.

❒❒ What are the therapeutic uses of atropine?

It is used in preoperative medication, in bradycardia, in ophthalmology to produce mydriasis, to reduce cholinergic hyperactivity. It is also used to treat Parkinsonism, as an antispasmodic, and in some OTC preparations for rhinitis and hay fever.

❒❒ What are the adverse effects of atropine?

Dry mouth, blurred vision, photophobia, tachycardia, GI distress and hot and dry skin.

❒❒ What other classes of drugs will interact with atropine and why?

Tricyclic antidepressants, phenothiazines, antihistamines and other drugs with anticholinergic properties.

❒❒ What groups of patients are very susceptible to atropine toxicity?

Children, especially infants, are very sensitive to the hyperthermic effects of atropine. Deaths have followed doses as small as 2 mg.

❒❒ How is atropine toxicity treated?

The drug should be removed from the stomach if possible. Overdoses are generally treated symptomatically using artificial respiration and cool packs. Physostigmine may be beneficial but most poison control experts now consider it more dangerous and no more effective than symptomatic management. If necessary, small doses can be given slowly.

❒❒ Which drug when applied to the skin in a transdermal patch is used to prevent or reduce the occurrence of nausea and vomiting associated with motion sickness?

Scopolamine.

❒❒ Which drugs block the action of acetylcholine and similar agonists at the nicotinic receptors of both parasympathetic and sympathetic autonomic ganglia?

Ganglionic blocking drugs like hexamethonium and tetraethylammonium, mecamylamine and trimethaphan.

❒❒ How are these ganglionic blockers used clinically?

In the treatment of hypertensive emergencies and to produce controlled hypotension.

❒❒ Why are they used very little if at all anymore?

There are more selective autonomic blocking agents available.

❒❒ What is another name for adrenergic agonists?

Sympathomimetics.

❑❑ **What types of sympathomimetics are there?**

Direct agents, indirectly acting agents, mixed agents and those that act reflexly by stimulation of alpha or beta adrenergic receptors in the circulation.

❑❑ **What is meant by the term indirect acting agent?**

A drug that acts as a result of releasing norepinephrine from the nerve ending.

❑❑ **Name two indirect acting adrenergic agonists?**

Tyramine and amphetamine.

❑❑ **What are the differences in location between α_1 and α_2 – adrenergic receptors?**

α_1 receptors are located on the effector organs postsynaptic membrane and α_2 receptors are predominantly located on the presynaptic membrane.

❑❑ **Epinephrine interacts with which receptor types?**

α_1, α_2, β_1 and β_2 – adrenergic receptors.

❑❑ **What organ systems does epinephrine exert its prominent effects on?**

The cardiovascular system (vasoconstriction of arterioles in the skin; viscera and mucus membranes) and the respiratory system. In addition it has certain metabolic effects such as increased glycogenolysis and release of glucagon and decreased release of insulin which results in hyperglycemia.

❑❑ **What are the cardiac effects of epinephrine?**

There is an increased heart rate and contractility.

❑❑ **What are the vascular effects of epinephrine?**

Cutaneous blood flow is reduced, renal blood flow is reduced, skeletal blood flow can be increased or decreased, and coronary blood flow is increased.

❑❑ **How is blood pressure effected by epinephrine?**

There is increased systolic pressure, decreased diastolic pressure and no change in mean pressure.

❑❑ **How is blood pressure effected by norepinephrine?**

There is increased systolic, diastolic and mean blood pressure.

❑❑ **What are the effects of epinephrine on the respiratory tract?**

There is bronchodilation.

❏❏ What are the ocular effects of epinephrine?

Epinephrine lowers intraocular pressure.

❏❏ What are the metabolic effects of epinephrine?

There is increased glycogenolysis and release of glucagon and decreased release of insulin resulting in hyperglycemia.

❏❏ How is epinephrine administered?

It is usually inhaled but also can be given SC.

❏❏ What are the adverse effects of epinephrine?

Cardiac arrhythmias, hypertension, palpitations, dizziness, anxiety, headache, tremor, myocardial infarction due to increased cardiac work and pulmonary edema.

❏❏ Why is epinephrine contraindicated in hyperthyroidism?

Hyperthyroid patients already are sensitized to sympathetic stimulation.

❏❏ What receptors does norepinephrine interact with?

α_1, α_2 and β_1 – adrenergic receptors but it has a stronger affinity for alpha receptors in comparison to beta adrenergic receptors.

❏❏ Describe the cardiovascular effects of norepinephrine?

Cardiac output is slightly decreased due to reflex effects and total peripheral resistance is increased

❏❏ What is the therapeutic use of norepinephrine?

In the treatment of shock.

❏❏ What receptors does isoproterenol interact with?

β_1 and β_2 – adrenergic receptors.

❏❏ What are the effects of isoproterenol on blood pressure?

The mean pressure decreases, systolic pressure increases and diastolic pressure decreases.

❏❏ What is the therapeutic use of isoproterenol?

Bronchodilation.

❏❏ What receptors does dopamine interact with?

Dopamine receptors (D_1), β_1 and α_1 – adrenergic receptors.

❑❑ Describe the vascular effects of dopamine?

It primarily dilates the renal and mesenteric vasculature.

❑❑ What effects does dopamine have on the kidney?

Renal blood flow increases, glomerular filtration rate is increased and sodium excretion is increased.

❑❑ What are the therapeutic uses of dopamine.

It is used to treat shock of various origins.

❑❑ What is dobutamine?

It is a dopamine analog.

❑❑ How is dobutamine used?

For the treatment of unstable congestive heart failure and shock.

❑❑ What effects does phenylephrine have on blood pressure?

Primarily vasoconstriction but the subsequent rise in blood pressure also leads to a reflex bradycardia.

❑❑ What are the therapeutic uses of phenylephrine?

It is a nasal decongestant and is also used to treat hypotension.

❑❑ What receptors does clonidine interact with?

α_2 – adrenergic receptors.

❑❑ What does clonidine do to the blood pressure?

It lowers blood pressure through an action in the CNS.

❑❑ What is the major mechanism of action for amphetamine?

It is an indirect acting amine, releasing novepinephrine, dopamine and serotonin.

❑❑ What effect does amphetamine have on the CNS?

It causes CNS stimulation and appetite suppression.

❑❑ What are the toxic effects of amphetamine?

Psychological and physical dependence, psychosis, confusion, insomnia, headache, restlessness, heart palpitations, tachycardia and impotence.

❒❒ What are the symptoms of the dependence produced by amphetamine?

Craving, prolonged sleep, general fatigue, hyperphagia and depression.

❒❒ What effects of amphetamine show tolerance?

The anorexigenic and mood improvement effects.

❒❒ Name two uses of amphetamine?

Attention deficit hyperactivity syndrome and narcolepsy.

❒❒ What receptors does phenylpropanolamine interact with?

α_1 - adrenergic receptors.

❒❒ What are the pharmacological effects of phenylpropanolamine?

It causes vasoconstriction and stimulation of the hypothalamic satiety center.

❒❒ What are the therapeutic uses of phenylpropanolamine?

It is used as a nasal decongestant and an appetite suppressant.

❒❒ Terbutaline and ritodrine interact with which receptors?

They are selective β_2 - adrenergic receptor agonists.

❒❒ What is the therapeutic use of terbutaline?

It is a bronchodilator used to treat asthma.

❒❒ What is the therapeutic use of ritodrine?

It is used to delay premature delivery.

❒❒ What is prazosin?

It is an alpha adrenergic receptor blocker.

❒❒ Which receptors does it interact with?

It interacts with and blocks the α_1 – adrenergic receptors.

❒❒ Explain the effects of prazosin on the cardiovascular (C.V.) system?

It causes vasodilation with little change in the heart rate.

❒❒ What are the side effects of prazosin?

Drowsiness, dizziness and headache.

❒❒ What is the first dose effect with prazosin?

There is marked postural hypotension with the first dose, therefore the drug should be taken at bedtime.

❒❒ How is prazosin used therapeutically?

It is used mainly to treat hypertension

❒❒ What is propranolol?

A nonselective beta adrenergic blocker.

❒❒ What receptors does propranolol interact with?

It causes competitive blockade of both β_1 and β_2 – adrenergic receptors. It has no intrinsic agonistic properties.

❒❒ The olol suffix on a drug means the drug is what?

The drug is a beta blocker.

❒❒ Describe the C.V. effects of propranolol?

The heart rate decreases, cardiac output decreases, oxygen consumption decreases, there is a slowly developing reduction in blood pressure and sinus rate is decreased as well as conduction is slowed.

❒❒ What are the metabolic effects of propranolol?

The normal rise in plasma free fatty acids associated with the beta response is inhibited and the hyperglycemic response to epinephrine is reduced.

❒❒ Does propranolol effect bronchial smooth muscle?

It increases the tone of bronchial smooth muscle and airway resistance is increased.

❒❒ What are the side effects of propranolol?

There is fatigue, lethargy, GI upset, wheezing and coldness in the extremities.

❒❒ What are the therapeutic uses of propanolol?

It is used to treat hypertension, hyperthyroidism, migraine headache, cardiac arrhythmias and angina pectoris.

❒❒ Name two other nonselective beta antagonists besides propranolol?

Timolol and nadolol

❑❑ What are the therapeutic uses of timolol and nadolol?

They are used for the treatment of glaucoma.

❑❑ What adverse effects are associated with the use of nonselective beta blockers?

Bradycardia, bronchoconstriction, they may hide the warning signs of hypoglycemia, fatigue, depression and sexual dysfunction.

❑❑ What is the mechanism of action of metoprolol?

It is a competitive blocker of beta$_1$ receptors with no agonist properties.

❑❑ What are the C.V. effects of metoprolol?

It inhibits the inotropic and chronotropic actions of the β_2 - adrenergic agonists and it reduces blood pressure

❑❑ What is metoprolol used for clinically?

Hypertension.

❑❑ What is timolol used for clinically?

To treat open angle glaucoma.

❑❑ What is the mechanism of action of timolol?

It is a nonselective beta adrenergic receptor blocker.

❑❑ What is the mechanism of action of phenoxybenzamine?

It is a noncompetitive α_1 and α_2 – adrenergic receptors blocker.

❑❑ How is phenoxybenzamine used clinically?

It is used for pheochromocytoma and benign prostatic hypertrophy.

❑❑ What are the toxicities associated with the use of phenoxybenzamine?

Postural hypotension, reflex tachycardia and nasal stuffiness.

❑❑ What is yohimbine?

A selective α_2 – adrenergic receptor antagonist.

❑❑ What is the therapeutic use of yohimbine?

It may have use in treating male sexual dysfunction.

❒❒ What do pindolol, labetalol, nadolol, acebutolol, bisoprolol, esmolol and atenolol have in common?

They are all beta adrenergic receptor blocking agents.

❒❒ What is methylphenidate?

An amphetamine variant whose major pharmacologic effects and abuse potential are similar to those of amphetamine. It is a mild CNS stimulant with more prominent effects on mental than motor activities.

❒❒ What is the therapeutic use of methylphenidate?

It is effective in treating attention deficit hyperactivity disorder and narcolepsy.

❒❒ What is the toxicity of methylphenidate?

Large doses produce signs of generalized CNS stimulation that may lead to convulsions. It shares the abuse potential of the amphetamines.

❒❒ What is the mechanism of action of ephedrine ?

It stimulates the release of norepinephrine from nerve terminals and also acts as a direct adrenergic agonist.

❒❒ How is ephedrine used clinically?

Hypotension, urinary incontinence and bronchospasm.

❒❒ What are the adverse effects of ephedrine?

Arrhythmias, palpitations, insomnia and hypertension.

❒❒ How is phentolamine used clinically?

Its major clinical use is in the management of pheochromocytoma.

❒❒ Name four selective β_1 - adrenergic receptor blockers?

Metoprolol, atenolol, esmolol and acebutolol.

❒❒ Is the selectivity of the beta blockers absolute?

No, it depends on the dose with selectivity being lost at higher doses.

❒❒ What are the main advantages of β_1 - adrenergic receptor selectivity?

They have selective effects on the heart without blocking the β_2 - adrenergic receptors in bronchial smooth muscle.

❑❑ Name two drugs that are β_1 –adrenergic receptor blockers but in addition have β_1 –adrenergic receptor agonistic properties?

Acebutolol and pindolol.

❑❑ How are acebutolol and pindolol used clinically?

For the treatment of hypertension in patients prone to bradycardia.

❑❑ What are the advantages of using acebutolol and pindolol?

They produce bronchoconstriction only at very high doses.

❑❑ What is the mechanism of action of guanethidine?

It blocks the release of stored norepinephrine after first entering the peripheral adrenergic nerve by a reuptake mechanism for norepinephrine and binding to storage vesicles.

❑❑ How is guanethidine used clinically?

It is used for the treatment of hypertension.

❑❑ What is the mechanism of action of reserpine?

It blocks norepinephrine transport from the cytoplasm into intracellular storage vesicles.

❑❑ What are the therapeutic uses of reserpine?

Hypertension.

❑❑ What are the adverse effects of reserpine?

CNS depression and bradycardia.

❑❑ Name three β_2 –adrenergic receptor agonists?

Albuterol, metaproterenol and terbutaline.

❑❑ What is the therapeutic use of the β_2 –adrenergic receptor agonists?

They are used mainly in the treatment of bronchospasm and asthma.

PHARMACOLOGY OF THE CENTRAL NERVOUS SYSTEM

ANALGESICS

❑❑ What is an analgesic?

A drug that relieves pain at a dose that has little or no effect on other body functions.

❑❑ How are analgesics classified?

By the severity of the pain that they relieve, by their ability to produce dependence and by their mechanism of action.

❑❑ What type of pain is easiest to deal with?

Acute pain.

❑❑ What are NSAIDs?

A group of dissimilar drugs with the same mechanism of action, that is inhibition of cyclooxygenase with subsequent inhibition of prostaglandin synthesis.

❑❑ Name four groups of NSAIDS?

Salicylates, indoleacetic acids, propionic acids, oxicams, fenamates and pyrazolones.

❑❑ What is the mechanism of action of the salicylates?

Inhibition of cyclooxygenase by acetylation. Cyclooxygenase is required for synthesis of prostaglandins and leukotrienes.

❑❑ How does the mechanism of action of aspirin differ from the other NSAIDS?

The effect of aspirin is irreversible, all the others are reversible inhibitors of cyclooxygenase.

❑❑ What are the main therapeutic uses of the nonsteroidal anti-inflammatory agents?

Anti-inflammatory agents, analgesics, antipyretics and antiplatelet agents.

❑❑ Why does blockade of prostaglandin synthesis relieve pain?

Prostaglandins convert pain receptors into a more sensitized form.

❑❑ What is the difference between COX-1 and COX-2 inhibitors?

COX-1 is constitutively expressed in most tissues and is thought to protect the gastric mucosa while COX-2 is expressed constitutively in the kidney and brain and can be induced at sites of inflammation. Thus inhibition of COX-2 may explain anti-inflammatory activity.

❑❑ Aspirin and the salicylates are primarily inhibitors of which isozymes?

COX-1 and COX-2 (at high concentration).

❑❑ How is aspirin metabolized?

It is converted to salicylate and then conjugated to glycine and glucuronides.

❑❑ What is the difference in aspirin metabolism between analgesic and antiinflammatory doses?

Conjugation occurs primarily at analgesic and antipyretic doses, while at antiinflammatory doses it is primarily excreted as salicylate. Excretion follows zero order kinetics.

❑❑ What are the main pharmacological actions of aspirin?

Analgesia, anti-inflammatory action, antipyresis and prevention of thrombus formation and prolongation of bleeding time.

❑❑ How does aspirin prevent thrombus formation and prolong bleeding times?

Aspirin shifts the balance between inhibition of prostacyclin formation in the vasculature and inhibition of aggregation of platelets to inhibition of aggregation thus increasing the bleeding time.

❑❑ What are the therapeutic uses of aspirin?

Analgesia, antipyresis, anti-inflammation, acute rheumatic fever, and rheumatoid arthritis.

❑❑ What are the adverse effects of aspirin on the GI tract?

GI irritation and bleeding, gastric ulceration and hemorrhage and exacerbation of peptic ulcers.

❑❑ Does aspirin have effects on the cardiovascular system?

Not at therapeutic doses but at large doses there is dilation of peripheral vessels and toxic amounts cause central vasomotor paralysis.

❑❑ What are the effects of aspirin on the respiratory system?

Low doses increase oxygen consumption and CO_2 production, higher doses stimulate the respiratory center directly resulting in respiratory alkalosis and then eventually respiratory paralysis and acidosis occur.

❏❏ How does aspirin effect acid-base balance?

These effects are related to the respiratory effects. Low doses increase CO_2 production. At higher doses there is compensation for respiratory alkalosis and at toxic doses there is metabolic acidosis. Also at toxic doses there are additional disturbances in potassium balance.

❏❏ What is salicylism?

Mild aspirin toxicity. It is characterized by ringing in the ears, dizziness, headache, mental confusion, deafness etc.

❏❏ What toxicities does aspirin have at very high doses?

CNS disturbances, GI disturbances, respiratory and acid-base balance disturbances.

❏❏ How do you treat overdose toxicity of aspirin?

Maintain respiration and circulation, minimize the amount of drug absorbed through gastric lavage and increase aspirin elimination by forced diuresis and alkalinization of the urine.

❏❏ Are allergic reactions common with aspirin?

They occur in about 1% of patients, with an increased incidence in asthmatics especially those with nasal polyps.

❏❏ What kind of drug interactions are associated with aspirin use?

It displaces other drugs from plasma protein binding sites thus increasing the effects of many drugs.

❏❏ Name two cox-2 inhibitors?

Celexoxib and rofexcoxib.

❏❏ What is the advantage of the COX-2 inhibitors over the salicylates?

They have fewer GI effects than the salicylates.

❏❏ What are the therapeutic uses of the COX-2 inhibitors?

Osteoarthritis, rheumatoid arthritis.

❏❏ What are the toxicities associated with the COX-2 inhibitors?

Abdominal pain, diarrhea, dyspepsia, edema in the lower extremities.

❏❏ What effect do the COX-2 inhibitors have on bleeding time?

They have little or no effect.

❏❏ What is the mechanism of action of the propionic acid derivatives?

They work the same as aspirin.

❏❏ How do the propionic acid inhibitors differ from aspirin in their GI effects?

They produce the same GI effects but to a lesser extent.

❏❏ What type of pain are the propionic acid inhibitors better used for than aspirin?

Dysmenorrhea

❏❏ Do the propionic acid inhibitors show cross-sensitivity to aspirin?

Yes they do.

❏❏ What is the advantage if any of naproxen over ibuprofen?

Naproxen is long acting and can be given twice daily.

❏❏ What is the advantage of ketoprofen?

It may be the best analgesic of the NSAIDS.

❏❏ How does acetaminophen differ from aspirin in its pharmacological actions?

It has little or no anti-inflammatory action.

❏❏ What is the mechanism of action of acetaminophen?

Inhibition of prostaglandin synthesis. It inhibits COX-1 and not COX-2. It may also possibly inhibit other isozymes of COX.

❏❏ How is acetaminophen metabolized?

By conjugation and oxidation by cytochrome P450 enzymes.

❏❏ How does acetaminophen effect the GI. Tract?

It has little or no effect.

❏❏ How does acetaminophen effect respiration or the acid base balance?

It has little effect.

❑❑ What are the therapeutic uses of acetaminophen?

It is used for analgesia and antipyresis, like aspirin.

❑❑ What are the adverse effects of acetaminophen?

They are generally mild and include skin rash, drug fever, and mucosal lesions.

❑❑ Does acetaminophen show cross sensitivity with the salicylates?

Yes.

❑❑ What types of long-term toxicity can occur with acetaminophen?

Hepatic damage.

❑❑ What is the mechanism of the acetaminophen hepatotoxicity?

Certain metabolites of acetaminophen bind to hepatic proteins and cause necrosis.

❑❑ What agent is used to treat acetaminophen overdose toxicity?

Sulfhydryl compounds such as N-acetylcysteine.

❑❑ What drugs are considered opioid analgesics?

Purified alkaloids from the opium poppy, semisynthetic derivatives of these alkaloids and a group of synthetic compounds with actions similar to the opiates.

❑❑ What are the general features of the opioids?

They have certain common structural features, they are stereospecific and they act at specific receptor sites.

❑❑ Which drug is considered the prototype and standard for the opioid drugs?

Morphine.

❑❑ What is the mechanism of action of morphine?

It is an agonist at specific receptors termed opiate receptors.

❑❑ What types of opiate receptors does morphine act on?

Mu, kappa and delta.

❑❑ What are the main pharmacological actions of morphine?

Analgesia, respiratory depression, drowsiness and sedation, euphoria and tranquility, pupillary constriction, nausea and vomiting, and GI effects.

❑❑ What type of analgesia does morphine produce?

It produces analgesia without loss of consciousness, it is more effective against continuous dull pain than sharp intermittent pain, and it acts at both the spinal level and at higher levels.

❑❑ What effect does morphine have on respiration?

It produces respiratory depression primarily due to a decrease in sensitivity in the chemoreceptor centers to plasma CO_2.

❑❑ What effect does morphine have on the eye?

It causes pupillary constriction.

❑❑ What effect does morphine have on the GI system?

Constipation is produced.

❑❑ Does morphine effect the cardiovascular system?

It has mild effects there such as orthostatic hypotension.

❑❑ How is morphine administered?

It can be given in many ways including IV, PO, SC or IM.

❑❑ Why are higher doses of morphine required orally?

Due to first pass metabolism.

❑❑ How is morphine metabolized?

It is mainly glucuronidated.

❑❑ Name two other important uses of morphine besides analgesia?

Sickle cell crisis and pulmonary edema due to acute left ventricular failure-dyspnea.

❑❑ What are the side effects of morphine use?

Dependence, increased pressure in the biliary tract, dysphoria and excitement, allergic reactions.

❑❑ What type of withdrawal symptoms are seen with use of the opiates?

It reflects an exaggerated rebound from the acute pharmacologic effects of the drug. The signs of withdrawal include rhinorrhea, lacrimation, yawning, chills, gooseflesh, hyperventilation, hyperthermia, mydriasis, muscular aches, vomiting, diarrhea, anxiety and hostility.

❑❑ **What are the major drug-drug interactions of morphine?**

It can interact with CNS depressants, antipsychotic agents and MAO inhibitors (antidepressants).

❑❑ **What are the contraindications for morphine use?**

Head injuries, decreased pulmonary function, pregnancy and urinary tract obstruction.

❑❑ **What are the two naturally occurring opiate alkaloids?**

Morphine and codeine.

❑❑ **Name two drugs that are opiate antagonists?**

Naltrexone and naloxone.

❑❑ **Name two drugs that are mixed opiate agonists/antagonists?**

Pentazocine, buprenorphine and butorphanol.

❑❑ **What two physiologic effects of morphine are not affected by tolerance?**

GI effects and pupillary constriction.

❑❑ **How does the potency of codeine compare to morphine?**

Codeine is about 1/10 as potent.

❑❑ **What are the therapeutic uses of codeine?**

Mild to moderate pain and cough suppression.

❑❑ **Is the abuse potential for codeine less or more than for morphine?**

Codeine has less abuse potential than morphine.

❑❑ **How do the effects of meperidine on the CNS compare with those of morphine?**

Meperidine may be excitatory at toxic doses or with chronic use.

❑❑ **How do the effects of meperidine on the GI tract compare with morphine?**

There is less constipation and less spasm of the biliary tract.

❑❑ **What effect does meperidine have on the eyes?**

Unlike most opiates it causes the pupils to dilate rather than constrict. This is related to its anticholinergic activity.

❑❑ **How is meperidine used clinically?**

It is used to produce analgesia.

❑❑ **What is the major difference in side effects of meperidine compared to morphine?**

Meperidine has fewer effects on the GI tract.

❑❑ **What drug interactions are involved with meperidine?**

Meperidine has very potent interactions with MAO inhibitors, tricyclic anti-depressants and chlorpromazine.

❑❑ **What happens if meperidine is given to patients taking MAO inhibitors?**

The combination may result in severe respiratory depression, hyperpyrexia and convulsions.

❑❑ **What is diphenoxylate?**

A drug related to meperidine that is a potent anti-diarrheal agent.

❑❑ **What is loperamide?**

It is also related to meperidine and is a potent anti-diarrheal agent.

❑❑ **What is fentanyl?**

It is a synthetic opioid and a meperidine analog. Fentanyl and its derivatives including sufentanil are the most potent opioid agonists available.

❑❑ **How is fentanyl used?**

It is a potent analgesic. It is also used to produce neuroleptoanalgesia and is used in cardiovascular surgery.

❑❑ **How is fentanyl administered?**

Either IV or transdermally or in lollipop form as preanesthetic medication for children.

❑❑ **What iare the main differences between methadone and morphine?**

In pharmacokinetic properties. For example, methadone is very effective and reliable when given orally. It also is longer acting than morphine. Tolerance and physiologic dependence develop more slowly with methadone than with morphine.

❑❑ **What are the uses of methadone?**

Analgesia and treatment of addiction.

❐❐ How does heroin differ from morphine?

Heroin is hydrolyzed into morphine and therefore has many properties similar to morphine. It is however, more lipid soluble and can get across the blood brain barrier faster.

❐❐ What is propoxyphene?

A compound structurally similar to methadone but with much weaker actions.

❐❐ How does propoxyphene compare as an analgesic to aspirin?

It is equianalgesic.

❐❐ Is propoxyphene addictive?

Its addictive properties are equivalent to codeine.

❐❐ What is a partial opioid agonist?

A compound that acts as an agonist when given alone but reduces or blocks the actions of full agonists such as morphine and may precipitate withdrawal in addicts.

❐❐ What are the therapeutic uses of pentazocine?

It is used to produce analgesia in cases of moderate to severe pain.

❐❐ What are the uses of buprenorphine?

Analgesia, treatment of opioid dependence, and treatment of cocaine abuse.

❐❐ How do opioid antagonists differ from opiate receptor agonists?

By slight alterations in structure, in their actions at opiate receptors and in their clinical uses.

❐❐ How does naloxone work?

It is an opioid receptor antagonist. It binds all opiate receptors to displace bound opioid agonists.

❐❐ How is naloxone used therapeutically?

To reverse the respiratory depression and coma of opioid overdose.

❐❐ What are the therapeutic uses of naltrexone?

It is useful for treating opioid dependence because it has a longer duration of action than naloxone.

❑❑ What are the adverse effects of naltrexone?

Hepatotoxicity, nausea, sedation and headache.

❑❑ What happens if naloxone or naltrexone is given in the absence of an opiate agonist?

Usually there is no physiologic effect in this situation.

❑❑ What opiates are useful as antitussive agents?

Dextromorphan and codeine.

❑❑ What is apomorphine?

A potent dopamine agonist used as an emetic agent. It is similar to morphine in structure.

❑❑ How do you treat an acute opioid overdose?

Support respiration and use naloxone.

DRUG USED TO TREAT HYPERURICEMIA AND GOUT

❑❑ What is hyperuricemia?

A condition in which the serum urate levels exceeds the serum solubility of monosodium urate. The serum is saturated at 7mg/100 ml.

❑❑ Why does hyperuricemia occur?

Through excessive uric acid synthesis or purine consumption, excessive purine synthesis, high dietary consumption of purines and/or tissue destruction or through diminished renal excretion.

❑❑ What conditions are prone to cause hyperuricemia?

Myeloproliferative symptoms, acute leukemia, multiple myeloma, polycythemia vera and aggressive chemotherapy or irradiation leading to tissue breakdown.

❑❑ What drugs may cause hyperuricemia?

Cytotoxic agents, ethambutol, pyrazinamide, cyclosporine, ethanol, nicotinic acid and salicylates at lower doses.

❑❑ Why do you want to treat hyperuricemia?

To prevent recurrent acute attacks of gout, to prevent tophaceous deposits from occurring, to allow the tophaceous deposits to dissolve and to prevent deposition of sodium urate crystals in the kidney.

❑❑ **When do you treat hyperuricemia?**

If symptoms of gout develop, if there is a family history of gout, if nephrolithiasis or renal failure are present, if there is an excretion of more than 1.1 gm. of uric acid/day or if the plasma uric acid levels are > 10 mg/dL in female or 13 mg/dL in males.

❑❑ **What drugs are used to treat hyperuricemia?**

Allopurinol and uricosuric drugs (probenecid and sulfinpyrazone).

❑❑ **What is the mechanism of action of allopurinol?**

Allopurinol inhibits the metabolism of hypoxanthine and xanthine to uric acid. As a consequence the plasma uric levels drop. Xanthine and hypoxanthine are more soluble than uric acid and are not nearly as likely to crystallize out of the plasma.

❑❑ **What is allopurinol metabolized to and what significance is that?**

It is metabolized principally to oxipurinol to which most of the pharmacological effect of allopurinol is due to.

❑❑ **What are the principal adverse reactions of allopurinol?**

GI irritation may occur occasionally and in addition drowsiness, headache and a metallic taste can occur.

❑❑ **What is the toxic syndrome associated with allopurinol use?**

It is a rare but serious effect and is associated with hypersensitivity reactions. Manifestations include rash and pruritus, GI distress, fever and hepatic and renal dysfunction.

❑❑ **What types of drug interactions are associated with allopurinol use?**

It inhibits the cytochrome P-450 enzymes that metabolize oral hypoglycemic agents and anticoagulants. It interferes with the normal metabolism of 6-mercaptopurine and it increases the toxicity of other cytotoxic agents like cyclophosphamide.

❑❑ **What are the major uses of allopurinol?**

Primary hyperuricemia, secondary hyperuricemia and to inhibit perfusion injury of tissues to be transplanted.

❑❑ **What therapeutic problems are associated with the use of allopurinol?**

The decrease in sodium urate levels may not be immediate and there may be an increase in the frequency of acute attacks of gout.

❑❑ **What is the mechanism of action of the uricosuric agents?**

At less than therapeutic doses they block tubular secretion of uric acid and at therapeutic doses they also block tubular reabsorption of uric acid.

❑❑ What are some of the therapeutic problems associated with use of the uricosuric agents?

There may be urate crystal formation in the kidney, plasma uric acid levels may only slowly decrease and there may be an increased frequency of acute attacks of gout.

❑❑ What are the contraindications of the uricosuric drugs?

A frequent recurrence of renal lithiasis, an excretion of more than 800 mg of uric acid/day and marked renal function impairment.

❑❑ What are the adverse effects of probenecid?

G.I distress, hypersensitivity reactions, headache, urinary frequency, hemolytic anemia, dizziness and flushing.

❑❑ What are the adverse effects of sulfinpyrazone?

Most frequent are abdominal pain and nausea, possible reactivation or exacerbation of peptic ulcers, and sulfinpyrazone inhibits thromboxane synthesis and platelet formation and is contraindicated in a patient with blood dyscrasias.

❑❑ What are the drug-drug interactions of probenecid and sulfinpyrazone?

They may inhbit the secretion of acidic organic drugs such as aspirin, penicillin and indomethacin. Probenecid will also retard the secretion of sulfinpyrazone. Sulfinpyrazone will displace oral hypolglycemic agents, warfarin and aspirin from plasma protein. Probenecid or sulfinpyrazone plus aspirin gives no uricosuric effect. Probenecid and sulfinpyrazone will speed up the excretion of oxypurinol and probenecid slows the clearance of naproxen by inhibiting hepatic metabolism.

❑❑ What are the drugs of choice for treating hyperuricemia?

Uricosuric agents are the first drugs of choice because they don't produce the severe toxic reactions occasionally seen with allopurinol. Allopurinol is the drug of choice when uric acid excretion is more than 800 mg per day., when the patient has renal insufficiency, when nephrolithiasis or large tophi are present and in preventing acute uric acid nephropathy in patients receiving cytolytic therapy for malignancy.

❑❑ What contributes to an attack of acute gout?

The exact cause is unknown but dietary stress, physical stress and emotional stress all play a role.

❑❑ What is the first choice drugs for an acute attack of gout?

Indomethacin, NSAIDS that don't produce hyperuricemia and colchicine. Only colchicine is specific for acute attacks.

❑❑ What is the mechanism of action of colchicine?

It binds to tubulin and prevents the formation of microtubules. It inhibits the migration of leukocytes into the joint and the phagocytosis of uric acid crystals. It also inhibits the release of the chemotactic factors and the glycoprotein, which causes joint pain and inflammation from the leukocytes.

❑❑ How is colchicine administered?

It can be given orally or I.V.

❑❑ What considerations should be taken into account when using colchicine?

If given orally, the therapeutic effect may occur at the same concentrations that cause GI distress. The sooner the drug is given after the attack starts the more effective the drug is. A full dose should not be repeated until two weeks have elapsed and use it with caution in patients with liver and/or kidney disease.

❑❑ What are the uses of colchicine?

It is used as a diagnostic aid for gout, to treat acute attack of gout when NSAIDS are contraindicated, and prophylactically to prevent recurring attacks.

❑❑ What are the adverse effects of colchicine?

Some initial signs associated with toxicity are burning of throat, abdominal pain, diarrhea, nausea, vomiting and hemorrhagic colitis. Side effects associated with overdose include anuria, alopecia, bone marrow depression and hepatocellular failure.

TREATMENT OF RHEUMATOID ARTHRITIS

❑❑ What is rheumatoid arthritis?

A chronic inflammatory disease with frequent acute attacks. The immune system is involved in attacking the joints and surrounding structures such as muscle tendons and most other connective tissue. There is inflammation of the synovial membrane.

❑❑ What is the purpose in treating rheumatoid arthritis?

To prevent pain, inflammation and joint destruction and to preserve joint mobility and to halt the disease process.

❑❑ What role do drugs have in the treatment of rheumatoid arthritis?

To relieve the symptoms and minimize the destruction caused by the inflammation.

❑❑ What drugs are used to treat rheumatoid arthritis?

Traditional approaches to treatment have included NSAIDS, disease modifying antirheumatic drugs (DMARDS) and corticosteroids. In recent years there has been a shift towards earlier use of aggressive treatment with DMARDS.

❑❑ Why are the COX-2 inhibitors useful in rheumatoid arthritis?

They provide pain relief with fewer GI problems than NSAIDS.

❑❑ What drugs are considered DMARDS?

Gold Salts, penicillamine, azathioprine, methotrexate, cyclosporine, etc.

❑❑ How do the gold salts work in the treatment of rheumatoid arthritis?

The mechanism of action is unknown but they directly affect inflammation. They don't inhibit prostaglandin synthesis.

❑❑ How are the gold salts administered?

Myochrisine and gold thioglucose are given I.M. while auranofin is taken orally.

❑❑ How are the gold salts used in the treatment of rheumatoid arthritis?

They are used early for non-responsive slow progressive disease.

❑❑ Do the gold salts work rapidly?

No, they take months to see effects.

❑❑ What are the side effects of the gold salts?

The most common effect is dermatitis. Also occurring are bone marrow depression and renal toxicity. Hepatitis and enteritis are rare Stomatitis and a metallic taste also may occur.

❑❑ How is methotrexate used in the treatment of rheumatoid arthritis?

It is finding increased use in the early stages of non-responsive or severe disease, and is now being used in the early stages of disease. Many rheumatolists consider it a first choice drug.

❑❑ What types of toxicity occur with methotrexate when it is used for the treatment of rheumatoid arthritis?

There is a dose related hepatotoxicity in 40% of patients treated and pulmonary toxicity may also occur.

❑❑ What is penicillamine?

It is a metabolite of penicillin and an analog of cysteine. The D form is used clinically.

❑❑ How is it used in the treatment of rheumatoid arthritis?

It is an effective alternative to gold therapy. It is used for patients with active, progressive erosive rheumatoid disease not controlled by conservative therapy.

❑❑ What type of toxicity is associated with the use of penicillamine?

Toxicity limits its usefulness. Proteinuria is encountered in 20% of patients. Immune complex nephritis has been seen in 4% of patients. Leukopenia and thrombocytopenia may occur at any time and may indicate aplastic anemia. Most deaths are due to aplastic anemia.

❑❑ How is sulfasalazine useful in arthritis?

Its mechanism is unknown. Either the 5-aminosalicylate or the sulfapyridine formed are the active forms.

❑❑ What are etanercept and infliximab?

Monoclonal antibodies. Etanercept is a soluble human TNF receptor and infliximab is an anti-TNF antibody.

❑❑ Why are etanercept and infliximab useful in the treatment of rheumatoid arthritis?

TNF is one cytokine that may play a role in the development of rheumatoid arthritis.

❑❑ What is Leflunomide?

A newer DMARD that reduces pyrimidine synthesis, thus decreasing rheumatoid inflammation.

BENZODIAZEPINES

❑❑ What classes of drugs are considered to be CNS depressants?

Benzodiazepines, barbiturates, alcohol and general anesthetics.

❑❑ What is the difference between sedation, hypnosis, and anesthesia?

Sedation is a decreased responsiveness to external stimuli but the person is not asleep. Hypnosis is a sleep like state from which the patient can be easily awakened and anesthesia refers to the situation where there is a state of unconsciousness where the patient is amnestic and unresponsive to pain or external stimuli.

❑❑ What is the difference in these drugs in the degree of depression produced?

Benzodiazepines produce sedation and hypnosis but they don't produce a true anesthetic state by themselves. The degree of CNS depression produced by barbiturates, alcohol and general anesthetics is dependent on the dose given. All three groups can produce all levels of CNS depression including depression of the respiratory centers and death.

❑❑ What is the common transmitter affected by all these CNS depressants?

GABA.

❑❑ What is the mechanism of action of the benzodiazepines?

They potentiate the action of GABA on the chloride channel to produce greater hyperpolarization than produced by GABA alone. They are not agonists and do not bind to the GABA sites on the $GABA_A$ receptor. They are sometimes referred to as positive allosteric modulators.

❑❑ What is the function of GABA in the CNS?

It is the major inhibitory transmitter in the CNS.

❑❑ What types of GABA receptors are there?

$GABA_A$, $GABA_B$ and $GABA_C$

❑❑ What are the differences between the three types of GABA receptors?

A is a ligand gated ion channel, with chloride ionophore; B is a G protein coupled receptor and C is a ligand gated ion channel, chloride ionophore and is located primarily in the retina.

❑❑ What is the function of the $GABA_A$ receptor?

It is the site of action of benzodiazepines, barbiturates, alcohol and general anesthetics.

❑❑ Which GABA receptor is the site of action of baclofen?

$GABA_B$.

❑❑ What is the mechanism of action of the barbiturates?

They bind to the barbiturate binding site on the $GABA_A$ receptor to potentiate action of GABA (positive allosteric regulator). They prolong the duration of action of GABA rather than intensify the GABA response. They also inhibit certain excitatory neurotransmitter receptors and have a general membrane depressant effect.

❑❑ What are the sites of action of ethanol?

Ethanol acts to decrease some voltage gated ion channels (e.g. Ca++ and K+); it also acts at some ligand gated ion channels ($GABA_A$ receptor) and inhibits some excitatory neurotransmitter receptors (NMDA glutamate). It also effects some G protein coupled receptors (opioid, noradrenergic and dopaminergic), signal transduction pathways (adenylate cyclase and protein kinase A and C) and has a general membrane depressant effect.

❑❑ What are the clinical uses of the benzodiazepines?

They are used for the treatment of anxiety, insomnia, epilepsy and seizures, sedation, amnesia and as preanesthetic medication. They are also used to produce muscle relaxation, and in alcohol and sedative-hypnotic withdrawal.

❑❑ What are the pharmacological effects of benzodiazepines on the CNS?

Decreased anxiety, hypnosis, muscle relaxation, anticonvulsant effects, anterograde amnesia and effects on learning and memory.

❑❑ Do the benzodiazepines have major effects on the cardiovascular system?

Their effects are minor except in severe intoxication. At preanesthetic concentrations there is decreased blood pressure and increased heart rate.

❑❑ What precautions must by taken when the benzodiazepines are given parenterally?

There may be irregular absorption from IM sites for some benzodiazepines. IV injections of diazepam may cause local pain and thrombophlebitis.

❑❑ After a single IV injection or single oral dose of benzodiazepines the duration of action is based on what?

Redistribution.

❑❑ After continuous daily usage of a benzodiazepine the duration of action is based on what?

Rate of metabolism.

❑❑ What is the primary means of elimination of the benzodiazepines?

Metabolism.

❑❑ How are the benzodiazepines metabolized?

The long acting benzodiazepines are metabolized by phase I and II reactions, while some of the short acting ones are metabolized solely by phase II conjugation.

❑❑ What effect does decreased hepatic function have on the benzodiazepines?

Generally decreased hepatic function results in decreased clearance rates of those drugs metabolized by oxidative pathways.

❑❑ Do the benzodiazepines induce drug metabolizing enzymes?

Not to any clinically significant degree.

❑❑ **What drugs might inhibit benzodiazepine drug metabolism?**

Cimetidine, oral contraceptives and isoniazid.

❑❑ **What common adverse effects are associated with benzodiazepine use?**

Drowsiness, sedation, impaired motor coordination, weakness, dizziness, confusion and memory loss all may occur.

❑❑ **Does tolerance develop to the effects of benzodiazepines?**

Tolerance develops to most of the adverse effects but with the antianxiety effects it develops much more slowly.

❑❑ **What happens upon withdrawal from the benzodiazepines?**

Increased anxiety, insomnia and CNS excitation, which may even progress to convulsions.

❑❑ **How does the intensity of withdrawal vary with the duration of action of the different benzodiazepines?**

It is less severe with the longer acting drugs since the CNS has a chance to gradually return to the normal state as the drug level gradually returns to zero.

❑❑ **What is meant by the term cross-dependence?**

Dependence to one drug in a class results in dependence to the other drugs in that class e.g. benzodiazepines.

❑❑ **What is buspirone?**

An antianxiety drug?

❑❑ **How does buspirone work?**

It is a partial agonist at the serotonin 5-HT_{1A} receptor.

❑❑ **How do the antianxiety effects of buspirone compare to the benzodiazepines?**

Buspirone relieves anxiety without causing marked sedative or euphoric effects.

❑❑ **How long does it take buspirone to work?**

It usually takes 1-2 weeks to produce antianxiety effects.

❑❑ **What are the side effects of buspirone?**

Tachycardia, palpitations, nervousness, gastrointestinal distress and paresthesias.

❒❒ **Can benzodiazepines be used in pregnancy?**

No, they have adverse effects on the fetus or newborn if used during pregnancy, delivery or breast -feeding. Concentration in the fetus is greater than in the mother.

❒❒ **What happens if benzodiazepines are given with other CNS depressants?**

The effects are additive.

❒❒ **What happens if benzodiazepine use is combined with alcohol?**

Fatalities may occur.

❒❒ **What is flumazenil?**

A benzodiazepine antagonist.

❒❒ **How does flumazenil work?**

It binds to the benzodiazepine site on the GABA receptor but has no effect on the chloride channel opening but prevents benzodiazepine from binding to the benzodiazepine site.

❒❒ **How is flumazenil used?**

It is used to reverse the sedative effect of benzodiazepines after anesthesia or sedation for brief surgical or diagnostic precedures. It is also used to reverse the effects of benzodiazepine overuse.

❒❒ **What would happen if flumazenil were given to someone dependent on benzodiazepines?**

It may precipitate a withdrawal reaction.

SEDATIVES AND HYPNOTICS

❒❒ **What are the CNS effects of the barbiturates?**

They depress the reticular activating system and alter normal sleep patterns.

❒❒ **What four barbiturates are used therapeutically?**

Thiopental, secobarbital, pentobarbital and phenobarbital.

❒❒ **Which barbiturate is best described as an ultra short acting one?**

Thiopental.

❒❒ **Name a long acting barbiturate?**

Phenobarbital.

❑❑ **What characteristics does increased lipid solubility provide to a barbiturate?**

With increased lipid solubility there is increased potency, increased metabolism, a faster onset of action and a shorter duration of action.

❑❑ **What effect do the barbiturates have on liver microsomal enzymes?**

They induce the liver microsomal drug metabolizing enzymes. Most induce these enzymes roughly 2 fold, but phenobarbital may increase them 6 fold.

❑❑ **Why is the duration of action of thiopental very short?**

As a result of redistribution of the drug from the brain.

❑❑ **What explains the long duration of action of phenobarbital?**

There is no redistribution but the long duration is based on the rate of metabolism and excretion. Since phenobarbital is eliminated slowly it has a very long half-life.

❑❑ **How can the rate of excretion of the barbiturates be increased?**

By alkalinization of the urine.

❑❑ **How do the barbiturates affect pain?**

They do not raise the pain threshold. They produce disorientation, restlessness, excitement and delirium in the presence of pain.

❑❑ **How do the barbiturates interact with other CNS depressants?**

They are additive with other CNS depressants.

❑❑ **Under what conditions are the barbiturates contraindicated?**

They are contraindicated in acute intermittent porphyria, in severe liver disease, and in cases of hypersensitivity to barbiturates and in uncontrolled pain.

❑❑ **Why are the barbiturates contraindicated in acute intermittent porphyria?**

The barbiturates induce the enzyme ALA synthetase, which will increase porphyrin synthesis.

❑❑ **What is the major sign of barbiturate toxicity?**

CNS depression, respiratory depression and depression of the thermoregulatory center.

❑❑ **How is barbiturate toxicity treated?**

By supporting respiration, supporting the cardiovascular system and by alkalinization of the urine.

❑❑ What is the mechanism of tolerance development to the barbiturates?

An increased rate of metabolism as well as adaptation of the CNS.

❑❑ Can withdrawal from barbiturates be fatal?

Yes.

❑❑ What are the common causes of insomnia?

Poor sleep hygiene, alcohol or caffeine intake, drug intake, psychological states such as anxiety and depression, sleep apnea, movement disorders, disorders of timing in the sleep wake pattern and various other medical conditions.

❑❑ What drugs are used to induce sleep?

Benzodiazepines, benzodiazepine agonists, barbiturates, antihistamines, antidepressants, anticholinergics, salicylates and some nonbenzodiazepine, nonbarbiturates (e.g. chloral hydrate)

❑❑ What are the reasons for using hypnotics?

They are used for several reasons including to shorten sleep onset, to prolong the duration of sleep, to reduce nocturnal wakefulness and to provide an anxiolytic effect during the next day when insomnia is accompanied by a marked element of anxiety.

❑❑ What do most hypnotics do on the first night of sleep?

Decrease sleep latency, lengthen the duration of sleep, decrease the awake time after sleep onset, decrease the number of awakenings, decrease delta sleep, REM sleep time, and stage II sleep time.

❑❑ What happens with chronic usage of hypnotics?

Tolerance develops, REM sleep time returns to normal, rebound insomnia and REM rebound.

❑❑ What pharmacokinetic principles must be taken into account when choosing a hypnotic?

The onset and duration of action of the hypnotic.

❑❑ What type of hypnotic is flurazepam?

It is a long acting hypnotic.

❑❑ What are the advantages of flurazepam?

Tolerance does not develop upon long term use, and it may be more effective on the second night than the first night. In addition REM rebound and rebound insomnia are not likely following discontinuation of chronic administration and it may have residual daytime antianxiety effects

❑❑ What are the disadvantages of flurazepam?

There may be residual daytime drowsiness.

❑❑ What is zolpidem?

A relatively new hypnotic that acts at the benzodiazepine binding site on $GABA_A$ but does not have the chemical structure of a benzodiazepine. It is an imidazopyridine derivative.

❑❑ What are the advantages of zolpidem?

It does not suppress REM sleep or delta sleep at therapeutic doses. The risk of tolerance and dependence with extended use is less than with the use of hypnotic benzodiazepines.

❑❑ What are the adverse effects of zolpidem?

Ataxia and confusion.

❑❑ Name an ultra-short acting hypnotic?

Triazolam

❑❑ What are the advantages of triazolam?

It has little residual daytime effects.

❑❑ What type of hypnotic is temazepam?

It is a benzodiazepine with a prolonged onset of action and a low incidence of daytime drowsiness.

❑❑ What are the contraindications to the use of hypnotics?

Sleep apnea syndrome, heavy uses of alcohol, pregnancy and if the patient needs nighttime alertness.

❑❑ What are the advantages and disadvantages of the antihistamines as hypnotics?

They can be purchased OTC. Overdoses can result in serious toxic effects including delirium, psychosis, and dystonic reactions particularly in the elderly. Tolerance develops to the hypnotic effects and they have anticholinergic effects as well as sedative and antihistamine effects.

ANTICONVULSANTS

❑❑ Define a seizure?

A seizure is an abnormal, synchronized, electrical depolarization of neurons in the CNS.

❑❑ What are the basic mechanisms of action of the anticonvulsant drugs?

They may limit sustained repetitive firing by blocking sodium channels, reduce voltage-sensitive calcium channel conductance, reduce glutamate-mediated excitation or enhance GABA mediated inhibition.

❑❑ What is the mechanism of action of phenytoin?

It binds to and prolongs the inactivated state of sodium channels.

❑❑ What are the clinical uses of phenytoin in epilepsy?

It is used for partial and generalized tonic/clonic seizures. It is also used for status epilepticus.

❑❑ Of what significance is the high degree of protein binding with phenytoin?

90% of the drug is bound to plasma proteins. This can reduce the amount of free drug present and only the free drug can pass through the blood brain barrier and be effective in epilepsy.

❑❑ What effect does phenytoin have on microsomal enzymes?

It is an inducer of microsomal enzymes and will increase the metabolism of concurrently administered drugs like oral contraceptives thus decreasing their effectiveness.

❑❑ What are the dose dependent adverse effects of phenytoin?

Nystagmus, diplopia, ataxia and lethargy.

❑❑ What are the idiosyncratic adverse effects of phenytoin?

Gingival hyperplasia, hirsutism, coarsening of facial features, drug rashes. lymphadenopathy, and mild peripheral neuropathy.

❑❑ Is phenytoin a teratogen?

It can produce the fetal hydantoin syndrome. Prenatal growth deficiency and mental deficiencies characterize this syndrome. There are also an increased number of congenital malformations such as cleft palate and heart malformations.

❑❑ What is fosphenytoin?

It is a prodrug of phenytoin.

❒❒ What are the advantages of fosphenytoin over phenytoin?

It has a neutral pH, it can be infused rapidly without pain or irritation, it can by mixed with dextrose solutions and it can be given IM if needed. No propyleneglycol or ethanol vehicle is needed.

❒❒ How is phenobarbital used in the treatment of epilepsy?

It is used to treat partial and tonic-clonic seizures especially in neonates and infants. It is also used to treat status epilepticus and febrile seizures.

❒❒ What are the chief pharmacokinetic features of phenobarbital?

There is slow but complete oral absorption, 50% protein bound and has a long half-life.

❒❒ What adverse effects are associated with the use of phenobarbital in epilepsy?

Sedation and mental dulling, paradoxical excitement in children and the elderly. There may also be drug rashes and possible dependence.

❒❒ What are the clinical uses of valproic acid?

It is a broad-spectrum antiepileptic agent. It is used in generalized tonic-clonic seizures, absence, myoclonic, atonic and partial seizures.

❒❒ What is the mechanism of action of valproic acid?

Its action probably results at least partially from an effect on sodium currents. It prolongs the inactivated state of sodium channels. It also increases GABA levels in the brain although the mechanism for this is unclear.

❒❒ What adverse effects are associated with the use of valproic acid?

The most common effects are GI complaints such as nausea and vomiting. It also produces tremor, hair loss, weight gain, rashes, hepatotoxicity and thrombocytopenia.

❒❒ What effect does it have on the offspring of women who take valproic acid during pregnancy?

The incidence of spina bifida is increased. There may also be an increased incidence of cardiovascular, orofacial and digital abnormalities.

❒❒ What effects do valproic acid have on liver microsomal metabolism?

It inhibits its own metabolism at low doses and it inhibits the metabolism of other drugs, especially the antiepileptic drugs phenobarbital and lamotrigine and prolongs their half-live and side effects.

❒❒ What is divalproex sodium?

A long acting preparation of valproic acid.

❑❑ **How is ethosuximide used in epilepsy?**

It is a first line drug used to treat absence seizures without tonic-clonic seizures. It is not good for grand mal epilepsy.

❑❑ **What is the mechanism of action of ethosuximide?**

Its mechanism probably involves calcium channels. It also inhibits Na^+/K^+ ATPase and inhibits GABA aminotransferase.

❑❑ **What are the adverse effects of ethosuximide?**

GI complaints such as pain, nausea and vomiting are most common. Also seen are headache, behavior changes, rashes and rarely hematologic dyscrasias.

❑❑ **What is the advantage of felbamate in the treatment of epilepsy?**

It is a broad spectrum antiepileptic drug.

❑❑ **What toxic effect has limited the use of felbamate in the treatment of epilepsy?**

There is a high incidence of aplastic anemia and and severe hepatitis.

❑❑ **How does gabapentin work?**

Its structure resembles GABA and it seems to increase the amounts of GABA.It appears not to act on GABA receptors, however, but may alter GABA metabolism or its nonsynaptic release.

❑❑ **What are the therapeutic uses of gabapentin?**

It is a useful adjunct drug for treating partial seizures and tonic-clonic seizures.

❑❑ **What are the adverse effects of gabapentin**

The most common adverse effects are somnolence, dizziness, ataxia, headache and tremor.

❑❑ **What are the uses for topiramate in epilepsy?**

It is an adjunct drug for treating partial and tonic-clonic seizures and shows promise in Lennox-Gastaut (complex multiple seizures) in children.

❑❑ **What are the adverse effects of topiramate?**

Somnolence, cognitive slowing and renal stones. It is teratogenic in animal models but no human fetal abnormalities have been noted.

❑❑ **What is the main use for benzodiazepines in epilepsy?**

To treat status epilepticus and occasionally for add-on use.

❑❑ Which benzodiazepines are preferred for the treatment of status epilepticus?

Diazepam and lorazepam.

❑❑ Why is the use of benzodiazepines limited in duration?

Tolerance soon develops, so they are not good for long-term use.

❑❑ How is lamotrigine used in the treatment of epilepsy?

It is used as adjunctive therapy for partial seizures and shows promise for tonic-clonic and Lennox-Gastaux (mixed seizures).

❑❑ What adverse effects are associated with the use of lamotrigine?

Rash, dizziness, headache, diplopia, nausea, and somnolence.

❑❑ For which group of anticonvulsants is it most useful to check drug levels?

The older established antiepileptics, as their therapeutic window is smaller.

❑❑ How is carbamazepine used in the treatment of epilepsy?

It is used to treat partial and tonic-clonic seizures. Its use is similar to phenytoin.

❑❑ How is carbamazepine metabolized?

It is metabolized by the liver to a 10,11 epoxide which contributes to its toxicity and adverse effects.

❑❑ Does carbamazepine affect liver microsomal enzymes?

It is a microsomal enzyme inducer, and can induce its own metabolism.

❑❑ What adverse effects are associated with the use of carbamazepine?

Nausea, diplopia, blurred vision, ataxia, rashes, bone marrow suppression and hyponatremia.

❑❑ What is oxcarbazepine?

A prodrug of 10-hydroxycarbazepine.

❑❑ What advantages does oxcarbazepine have over carbazepine?

It is more tolerable, doesn't induce its metabolism, and has less protein binding and possible fewer allergic reactions.

ANTIPARKINSONISM DRUGS

❐❐ What are the prominent symptoms of Parkinson's disease?

Tremor, akinesia or bradykinesia, rigidity and loss of normal postural reflexes.

❐❐ What is the basic pathology of parkinson's disease?

There is a degeneration of the nigrostriatal dopamine neurons.

❐❐ What is the major drug used to treat Parkinson's disease?

Levodopa

❐❐ How does levodopa work in the treatment of Parkinson's disease?

It bypasses the rate-limiting step in dopamine synthesis. It provides a substitute source of dopamine. It utilizes an enzyme, aromatic amino acid decarboxylase that is found in many cell types.

❐❐ What are the side effects of levodopa?

G.I (e.g. nausea), peak dose dyskinesia, cardiovascular problems, behavioral problems and sleep disturbances.

❐❐ What drug interactions are associated with levodopa?

Vitamin B6 may prevent its therapeutic effects. Combinations with monamine oxidase A inhibitors can lead to hypertensive crises.

❐❐ What are the limitations to the use of levodopa?

On-off phenomenon, interaction with vitamin B6, and concurrent use of monamine oxidase.

❐❐ What is meant by the on-off phenomenon?

Fluctuations or rapid changes in clinical response. The plasma levels of levodopa may drop quickly and this may cause sudden immobility and tremors.

❐❐ What is the advantage of using drug free holidays when using levodopa?

They may alleviate some of the neurological and behavioral adverse effects of levodopa.

❐❐ What are the advantages of using carbidopa in the treatment of Parkinson's disease?

It is an aromatic amino acid decarboxylase inhibitor potentiating the action of levodopa. It does not cross the blood brain barrier so its effects are peripheral. It reduces many of the side effects of levodopa and allows the use of lower doses of levodopa.

❑❑ How is carbidopa used in Parkinson's disease?

In combination with levodopa.

❑❑ Name two dopamine agonists used to treat Parkinson's disease?

Bromocriptine, pergolide, pramipexole and ropinirole.

❑❑ How do dopamine agonists work to treat Parkinson's disease?

They are direct dopamine receptor agonists (bromocriptine D_2 and pergolide D_1 and D_2)

❑❑ How do pramipexole and ropinirole differ from bromocriptine and pergolide?

These newer agents are non-ergots and avoid some ergot-associated side effects.

❑❑ What are the adverse effects of bromocriptine and pergolide?

Similar to levodopa, nausea and vomiting, hallucinations, delirium, cardiac arrhythmias, postural hypotension and eryhthromelalgia.

❑❑ How are bromocriptine and pergolide used in the treatment of Parkinson's disease?

They are used primarily in combination with levodopa, allowing reduction in levodopa dosage. Bromocriptine can be used alone or in combination.

❑❑ What is the mechanism of action of selegiline?

It is monamine oxidase inhibitor, type B>>A. It reduces the metabolism of levodopa and dopamine thus enhancing and prolonging the antiparkinsonian effect of levodopa, thus allowing its dose to be reduced.

❑❑ How can selegiline be used in Parkinson's disease?

It is useful with levodopa to reduce motor fluctuations, especially end-of-dose wearing off. It is of little use in advanced disease.

❑❑ What are the adverse reactions of selegiline?

It can cause insomnia, a caffeine like buzz, atrial fibrillation and it may increase the side effects of levodopa.

❑❑ What is the rationale behind using catechol methyl transferase inhibitors (COMT inhibitors) in Parkinson's disease?

They block levodopa metabolism by COMT in the periphery and enhance the effectiveness of levodopa.

❑❑ Name two COMT inhibitors that have been approved?

Tolcapone and entacapone.

❑❑ What toxicity is associated with tolcapone that will probably limit its use?

Liver toxicity

❑❑ What is the rationale behind using anticholinergics in Parkinson's disease?

They shift the dopamine-acetylcholine balance by lowering cholinergic levels.

❑❑ What two drugs in this category have been used as antiparkinson's agents?

Benztropine and trihexyphenidyl.

❑❑ What are the side effects of benztropine and trihexyphenidyl?

They are atropine like and include dry mouth, blurred vision, constipation, urinary retention, memory impairment and psychosis.

❑❑ How does the efficacy of the anticholinergics compare to levodopa?

They are much less efficacious than levodopa and are usually used just as adjuvants in parkinsonian therapy.

❑❑ Why is amantadine used in the treatment of Parkinson's disease?

It was found to modestly reduce tremor, rigidity and bradykinesia in about two-thirds of Parkinson's disease patients.

❑❑ What is the mechanism of action of amantadine in Parkinson's disease?

Its mechanism of action is basically unknown, but it may be a glutamate receptor antagonist. It may also enhance the release of dopamine form surviving nigral neurons or inhibit the reuptake of dopamine.

❑❑ What two drugs may inhibit the progression of Parkinson's disease?

Selegeline and vitamin E

❑❑ How do selegiline and vitamin E work to halt progression of Parkinson's disease?

They may decrease the production of toxins or free radicals.

DRUG ABUSE AND DEPENDENCE

❑❑ What is meant by the term drug abuse?

The inappropriate and usually excessive self-administration of a drug for nonmedical purposes in a manner that is harmful to the individual and/or society.

❒❒ **What is drug dependence?**

A situation that includes elements of physical dependence and withdrawal, habituation/tolerance and psychological dependence (craving for the drug).

❒❒ **Is caffeine addicting?**

With caffeine, dependence and withdrawal occur and there is anxiety, muscle tension and headaches. Lethargy and irritability also may occur.

❒❒ **What pharmacological sites does nicotine effect?**

It is a nicotinic cholinergic agonist with the CNS being the most important site of action

❒❒ **What effects are seen after taking nicotine?**

There is transient stimulation followed by a more persistent depression. There is psychological stimulation, relaxation, stimulation (increased respiration, tremors, and convulsions), depression at toxic doses and vomiting. There is also increased heart rate and blood pressure, and increased tone and motor activity, nausea and vomiting.

❒❒ **What is a fatal dose of nicotine?**

The fatal dose is 60 mg in an adult.

❒❒ **How is nicotine toxicity treated?**

Vomiting should be induced or use gastric lavage and supportive therapy.

❒❒ **What are the components in tobacco smoke responsible for the adverse effects after chronic use?**

Carbon monoxide, nitrogen oxides, nicotine, ammonia, nitrosamines, hydrogen cyanide, hydrocarbons, alcohols, aldehydes, ketones and tar (polycyclic aromatic hydrocarbons).

❒❒ **What are the adverse effects of tobacco smoke?**

Cardiovascular disease, neoplastic disease, chronic obstructive pulmonary disease, abortion or low birth weight infants and pulmonary dysfunction in exposed non-smokers.

❒❒ **What are the signs of nicotine withdrawal?**

The following signs are part of the nicotine withdrawal syndrome: irritability, impatience, hostility, anxiety, dysphoria or depressed mood, difficulty concentrating, restlessness, decreased heart rate, and increased appetite or weight gain.

❒❒ **How is nicotine withdrawal treated?**

Nicotine replacement therapy (nicotine supplements) alleviates the withdrawal syndrome. Clonidine has been used but is an investigational agent at present. It reduces central noradrenergic activity. Bupropion has also been used.

❏❏ What are the symptoms of alcohol withdrawal?

Alcohol withdrawal symptoms classically consist of hyperexcitability in mild cases and convulsions, toxic psychosis and delirium tremens in severe cases. The dose, rate, and duration of alcohol consumption determine the intensity of the withdrawal syndrome.

❏❏ How is alcohol withdrawal treated?

The major objective is to prevent seizures, delirium, and arrhythmias. Drugs such as chlordiazepoxide and clonidine are useful.

❏❏ What are the symptoms of opiate withdrawal?

There is a whole series of symptoms including craving, anxiety, lacrimation, rhinorrhea, yawning, sweating, restless sleep, pupil dilation, anorexia, goose flesh, irritability and tremor. At the peak there is nausea, vomiting, weakness, intestinal cramps and diarrhea. Heart rate and blood pressure are elevated and dehydration and disturbance of acid-base balance also occur.

❏❏ Is opiate withdrawal life threatening?

Usually not, except for people in really poor health.

❏❏ What drug alleviates the withdrawal symptoms from opiates?

Clonidine.

❏❏ How is opioid dependence treated pharmacologically?

There are several approaches. For clinically induced dependence the dose can be tapered to zero. For more serious dependence the patient can by stabilized on methadone and then it is withdrawn by tapering the dose, or by precipitated withdrawal or indefinite maintenance. Another approach is to put the patient on buprenorphine, a partial agonist. Then it is withdrawn with one of the schedules as with methadone. A third approach is to withdraw the drug either by straight withdrawal, or facilitated withdrawal with the aid of clonidine or an antagonist like naloxone or naltrexone.

❏❏ How does cocaine work?

It blocks dopamine uptake in the reward centers of the brain.

❏❏ What pharmacological effects does cocaine have?

There is elevation of mood, a reduction in the sense of fatigue, decreased performance caused by sleep deprivation and a toxic syndrome similar to that of amphetamine.

❏❏ What are the symptoms of cocaine withdrawal?

There is depression (cocaine blues) and craving.

❒❒ What drug is used to treat cocaine withdrawal?

Buprenorphine is an investigational agent that is used, as it is easier to withdraw from than cocaine.

ANTIPSYCHOTICS

❒❒ How are antipsychotics used clinically?

They are used primarily in the management of patients with psychotic or other serious psychiatric illnesses marked by agitation and impaired reasoning.

❒❒ Do the antipsychotics cure the disease?

No, they are palliative but do not cure the disease.

❒❒ What is another name for antipsychotic drugs?

Neuroleptics.

❒❒ What is the major factor that limits the use of the antipsychotics?

They have serious adverse effects.

❒❒ Do the antipsychotics have other uses beside psychosis?

They have a limited number of other uses including uses as antiemetics, for intractable hiccups and as pre-anesthetics.

❒❒ What determines which specific antipsychotic drug is used?

The specific drug used depends on patient characteristics such as age, coexisting medical problems, and other medications being taken and cost issues.

❒❒ What types of symptoms do the anti-psychotics work best against?

Positive symptoms such as delusions, thought disorders perceptual disturbances, inappropriate affects and increased motor function.

❒❒ Which antipsychotic is often given in the emergency room or the ICU for agitation?

Haloperidol or risperidol.

❒❒ What are the major groups of antipsychotic drugs?

Phenothiazines (e.g. chlorpromazine, perphenazine); thioxanthenes (e.g. thiothixene); butyrophenones (e.g. haloperidol); other heterocyclic compounds (e.g.clozapine, molindone, risperidone).

❑❑ What is the mechanism by which antipsychotics work?

These drugs block various receptors but their antipsychotic action is believed to be a result of dopamine receptor blockage, particularly postsynaptic D2 dopamine receptors. Some of the newer antipsychotics also block serotonin receptors. Other dopamine receptors also may play a role.

❑❑ How long do these antipsychotics take to demonstrate a positive effect?

Usually 2-3 weeks are required to show an obviously positive effect in a hospitalized patient. Chronically psychotic patients may take 6 weeks to 6 months for maximum benefits.

❑❑ What accounts for the multiplicity of side effects associated with these drugs?

Blockage of other receptors e.g. other dopamine receptors, serotinergic receptors, cholinergic, adrenergic and histaminergic receptors.

❑❑ What are the pharmacological effects of the antipsychotics?

In low doses operant behavior is reduced but spinal reflexes are unchanged. Exploratory behavior is diminished and responses to a variety of stimuli are fewer, slower, and smaller in magnitude, although the ability to discriminate stimuli is retained. Conditioned avoidance behaviors are selectively inhibited, whereas unconditioned escape or avoidance responses are not. Spontaneous motor activity in animals and in humans is diminished. They tend to normalize sleep disturbances characteristic of many psychoses. They impair vigilance in human subjects performing a variety of tasks.

❑❑ Are the antipsychotic drugs addicting?

They are not addicting by the usual definition, but some degree of physical dependence may occur with malaise and difficulty in sleeping developing several days after abrupt discontinuation. Tolerance develops to the sedative effects of neuroleptics over a period of days or weeks.

❑❑ What pharmacokinetic properties are shared by most antipsychotic drugs?

Lipophilicity, extensive protein binding, hepatic metabolism with formation of multiple metabolites and renal excretion. Oral preparations undergo first pass metabolism.

❑❑ How are the antipsychotics administered?

Orally, parenterally and with depot parenteral preparations.

❑❑ What is the role of clozapine in treating psychosis?

It is used for the treatment of refractory psychosis, psychosis in Parkinson's disease, and psychosis with tardive dyskinesia.

❑❑ What are the unique side effects of clozapine?

Agranulocytosis, elevated temperature and sialorrhea.

❑❑ When are depot forms of haloperidol and fluphenazine used?

For noncompliant patients with schizophrenia.

❑❑ What is the mechanism of the sedation associated with use of the antipsychotics?

Blockade of the α_1 – adrenergic receptors.

❑❑ Which group of antipsychotics is most likely to show sedation?

The low potency phenothiazines e.g. chlorpromazine.

❑❑ Which group of antipsychotics is most likely to produce seizures?

The lower potency phenothiazines.

❑❑ What extrapyramidal side effects are associated with the use of the antipsychotic drugs?

Akathisia, dystonia, parkinsonism and tardive dyskinesia.

❑❑ What group of antipsychotics are most likely to produce these extrapyramidal effects?

The high potency agents e.g. tricyclic piperazines (perphenazine, trifluoperazine and fluphenazine) and buytyrophenones.

❑❑ What is acute dystonia?

It is often seen with the initiation of antipsychotic drug therapy particularly with agents of high potency and may present as spasm of the muscles in the tongue, face, neck and back and may mimic seizures.

❑❑ How is dystonia treated?

It responds to anticholinergic antiparkinsonian drugs.

❑❑ What is akathisia?

It refers to strong subjective feelings of distress or discomfort (motor restlessness)?

❑❑ How is akathisia treated?

By reducing the dosage or changing the drug. Benzodiazepines or propranolol may help also.

❑❑ What is the mechanism of the drug induced parkinsonism?

It results from blockade of dopaminergic receptor sites in the striatum.

❑❑ **How is the drug induced parkinsonism treated?**

With oral anticholinergic agents.

❑❑ **What is the neuroleptic malignant syndrome?**

A rare disorder that resembles a very severe form of parkinsonism with catatonia, fluctuations in the intensity of coarse tremor and unstable blood pressure. Hyperthermia and diffuse muscular rigidity also characterize it. The prevalence is higher with relatively high doses of the more potent agents especially when they are given parenterally.

❑❑ **What is tardive dyskinesia?**

A late appearing neurological syndrome associated with the use of these drugs. It occurs more frequently in older patients, and risk may be greater in patients with mood disorders than in those with schizophrenia. It is characterized by stereotyped, repetitive, painless, involuntary, quick choreiform (ticlike) movements of the face, eyelids, mouth, tongue, extremities or trunk.

❑❑ **How is tardive dyskinesia treated or prevented?**

Prescribing neuroleptics at their lowest possible doses, providing drug free holidays and avoiding the simultaneous and prophylactic usage of anticholinergic agents. Overall prevention is very important, as treatment is usually unsatisfactory.

❑❑ **Which is more potent haloperidol or chlorpromazine?**

Haloperidol

❑❑ **Which of the two drugs produces more extrapyramidal reactions?**

Haloperidol.

❑❑ **What neuroendocrine side effects can result from use of the antipsychotics?**

Hyperprolactinemia, sexual dysfunction and weight gain.

❑❑ **Which of the antipsychotic drugs have cardiac effects?**

Chlorpromazine and thioridazine have direct effects on the heart as well as indirect actions through the CNS and autonomic reflexes.

❑❑ **What is risperidone?**

It is an antipsychotic in the group of other heterocyclics. It has greatly reduced side effects compared to haloperidol and chlorpromazine and is better tolerated by patients. It also may improve cognitive function and alleviate positive symptoms of schizophrenia better than cloassical antipsychotics.

❏❏ What types of drug interactions are associated with the antipsychotic agents?

The phenothiazines and thioxanthenes especially those of low potency affect the actions of a number of other drugs, sometimes with important clinical consequences. These include potentiation of central depressants such as general anesthetics, alcohol, sedatives and hypnotics, antihistamines and cold remedies. There is enhanced neurotoxicity in combination with lithium. Chlorpromazine increases the miotic and sedative effects of morphine and may increase its analgesic actions. It also markedly increases the respiratory depression produced by meperidine and other opioids. Sedatives or anticonvulsants that induce microsomal drug metabolizing enzymes can enhance the metabolism of antipsychotic agents, sometimes with significant clinical consequences. SSRIs including fluoxetine compete for hepatic oxidases and can elevate circulating levels of neuroleptics.

ANTIDEPRESSANTS

❏❏ What is depression?

A syndrome with a cluster of symptoms that includes mood and also vegetative, cognitive, impulse control, behavioral and somatic features. With depression there are changes in mood as opposed to thought disorders.

❏❏ What are some of the risk factors for depression?

Its peak onset is at 20-40 years of age. It is twice as likely to occur in women than men and is higher for the separated or divorced.

❏❏ What is the origin of depression?

It is a biologically based disease involving alterations in brain chemistry.

❏❏ What is the biogenic amine theory of depression?

Depression is due to a deficiency of monamine neurotransmitters notably norepinephrine (NE) and serotonin at certain sites in the brain.

❏❏ What are the sites of at which the antidepressant drugs act at in the CNS?

Certain metabolic enzymes like monamine oxidase, neurotransmitter uptake pumps and neurotransmitter receptors.

❏❏ What is the neurotransmitter receptor hypothesis of depression?

Abnormalities in the function of monamine neurotransmitter receptors leads to depression. Receptor disturbances may be caused by monamine neurotransmitter depletion. Depletion of neurotransmitters in depression leads to compensatory up-regulation of post-synaptic receptors and restoration of neurotransmitter levels by antidepressant therapy leads to a return to normal receptor levels. This hypothesis accounts for the delay in therapeutic effects of antidepressants and is also consistent with the direct receptor effects of some antidepressants.

❑❑ Are alterations in monamine transmission the only cause of depression?

Although they play a major role in the etiology of depression and mania they are unlikely to be the sole causative factor.

❑❑ How long does it take to obtain a therapeutic effect with the antidepressant drugs?

Pharmacological effects are immediate, but therapeutic effects take several weeks.

❑❑ What neurotransmitter receptors are involved in depression?

Certain postsynaptic receptors especially the 5HT2A receptor and the β_2, α_1 and α_2 - adrenergic receptors. In addition certain autoreceptors (those that recognize their own neurotransmitter) may be involved.

❑❑ What is the treatment strategy for depression?

Acute treatment, continuation and maintenance.

❑❑ What patients need maintenance treatment?

Those with severe and/or persistent symptoms and those with significant impairment and those with a family history or recurrence.

❑❑ What are the uses for the antidepressants?

For patients with depression, panic disorders, obsessive-compulsive disorders, enuresis and chronic pain.

❑❑ What are the different categories of antidepressant drugs?

Monamine oxidase inhibitors (MAOs), tricyclic antidepressants, heterocyclic antidepressants and selective serotonin reuptake inhibitors.

❑❑ What are the major MAO inhibitors used as antidepressants?

Phenelzine and tranylcypromine.

❑❑ What is their mechanism of action?

They are irreversible enzyme inhibitors that bind to MAO and destroy its function. They are not selective between MAO-A and MAO-B. MAO-A is the amine oxidase primarily responsible for norepinephrine, serotonin, and tyramine metabolism. Irreversible block of MAO, characteristic of the older inhibitors, allows significant accumulation of tyramine and loss of the first pass metabolism that protects against tyramine in foods. As a result the irreversible inhibitors are subject to a very high risk of hypertensive reactions to tyramine ingested. The reversible short acting inhibitors appear to be relatively free of this interaction.

❒❒ What are the immediate and chronic effects of the monamine oxidase inhibitors?

Their immediate biochemical effect is to block NE and 5HT breakdown in synaptic terminals and increase neurotransmitter release. Their chronic effect after 2-4 weeks is a positive effect on mood correlating to the down regulation of adrenergic receptors and feedback regulation that reduces synthesis of neurotransmitters.

❒❒ What is the role of the MAO inhibitors in antidepressive therapy?

They are no longer first line antidepressants. Although they are effective they have complex, unpredictable and often severe interactions with many food-derived amines and drugs making their use difficult and potentially dangerous.

❒❒ What are the preferred uses of the MAO inhibitors?

For atypical depression (weight gain, hypersomnia, and mood reactivity); for refractory cases and with depression associated with panic attacks.

❒❒ What are the adverse effects of the MAOIs?

Most of the adverse effects are related to MAO inhibition although some result from other mechanisms. There is orthostatic hypotension due to sympathetic block (bradycardia, decreased vasoconstriction and hypotension). There are also anticholinergic effects, CNS hyperstimulation or sedation and sexual dysfunction, weight gain and headache. Hepatic and hematologic dysfunctions occur rarely.

❒❒ What types of drug and food interactions occur with the monamine oxidase inhibitors?

Sympathomimetic drugs and tyramine containing foods may cause a hypertensive crisis. Anticholinergics, hypotensive drugs and CNS depressants especially meperidine may have their effects potentiated by these compounds. They may inhibit the detoxification of a number of centrally acting agents and they may enhance the hypoglycemic responses in patients receiving insulin or sulfonylurea hypoglycemics.

❒❒ What is the role of the tricyclic antidepressants (TCAs) in therapy?

They are effective antidepressants. They are preferred over the monoamine oxidase inhibitors as they lack dangerous food and drug interactions. Their use is accompanied by unwanted effects that limit patient compliance and an overdose can be lethal due to cardiovascular effects.

❒❒ Name two tricyclic antidepressants?

Amitriptyline, imipramine, clomipramine and doxepin.

❒❒ What is the mechanism of action of the tricyclic antidepressants?

They are reuptake inhibitors of sertonin and norepinephrine and to a lesser extent dopamine. They show varying degrees of selectivity and potency for norepinephrine and serotinin reuptake pumps. They also block muscarinic, cholinergic, histaminergic and α_1-adrenergic receptors.

❑❑ How long does it take to see an effect with the tricyclics?

Although uptake is inhibited quickly, clinical effects require several weeks.

❑❑ What is the most common adverse effect associated with the tricyclic antidepressants?

Anticholinergic effects (dry mouth, constipation, blurred vision, drowsiness, urinary hesitation, tachycardia, memory loss and confusion and delirium at higher doses).

❑❑ What are the other adverse effects associated with the tricyclic antidepressants?

They have a high incidence of side effects and a narrow therapeutic index limiting their use in some patient groups. Sedation and weight gains occur. Also seen are orthostatic hypotension, dizziness, drowsiness, sexual dysfunction, seizures and tremor.

❑❑ What is the biggest problem in using the antidepressants?

They are extremely dangerous when taken in overdose quantities and depressed patients are more likely than others to be suicidal. Cardiotoxicity and conduction delay may occur especially in overdose. Other dangerous toxicities include seizures, bowel and bladder paralysis, respiratory depression and coma with shock and occasionally metabolic acidosis.

❑❑ What typse of drug interactions are associated with the tricyclic antidepressants?

Use of alcohol may lead to greater than expected impairment of driving ability. Many other medications have the ability to increase or decrease tricyclic antidepressant levels. Patients who are prescribed tricyclic antidepressants with other medications should be monitored closely. Tricyclics potentiate the effects of biogenic amines and block the effects of indirectly acting amines (e.g. tyramine). Tricyclics also reverse the antihypertensive effects of some drugs e.g. guanethidine, methyldopa and clonidine.

❑❑ What are the clinical uses of the tricyclic antidepressants?

Severe depression, chronic pain, migraine, posttraumatic stress and enuresis in children.

❑❑ Which drugs are considered selective serotonin reuptake inhibitors (SSRIs)?

Currently five are available. Fluoxetine, sertraline, paroxetine,fluvoxamine and citalopram.

❑❑ What are the advantages of this class of antidepressants?

They have greater safety and tolerability compared to other classes of antidepressants. Patient compliance is increased and long term treatment has been shown to decrease relapse. They also have proven efficacy in many disorders.

❑❑ What is the mechanism of action of the SSRIs?

They selectively block reuptake of serotonin. There is little effect on norepinephrine and dopamine uptake.

❑❑ What are the main pharmacokinetic features of this group of drugs?

They have good absorption when given orally, a long half-life (especially fluoxetine), metabolism in the liver and excretion in the urine.

❑❑ What are the clinical indications of the SSRIs?

The treatment indications vary with the individual drugs. All of the selective reuptake inhibitors except fluvoxamine are indicated for the treatment of major depressive disorders. Sertraline and paroxetine carry indications for major depression, panic disorder and obsessive-compulsive disorder. Paroxetine has also been used for social phobia. Sertraline is also indicated for post traumatic stress and fluoxetine for premenstrual dysphoria. . Citalopram is indicated only for major depression.

❑❑ How do the various SSRIs vary in their clinical efficacy?

They are generally considered to be equally effective for the treatment of depression.

❑❑ What are the adverse effects of the selective serotonin uptake inhibitors?

For the most part they have fewer adverse effects than most other classes of antidepressants. Adverse effects include asthenia/fatigue, anxiety, insomnia, somnolence, tremor, GI symptoms, rashes, decreased libido, sexual dysfunction and headache.

❑❑ What is the risk of overdose with the SSRIs?

The risk is low (1/1,000,000) and toxicity rarely results in seizures or serotonin syndrome.

❑❑ What is the danger of overdose of the SSRIs?

A few deaths have occurred during overdosage when other drugs were also being taken. The likelihood of fatalities is very low.

❑❑ What type of drug interactions occurs with this group of drugs?

Some SSRIs are potent inhibitors of CYP 450 isoenzymes (especially fluvoxamine) and there may be interactions with other drugs metabolized by the cytochrome P450 system. There may be interactions between fluoxetine/sertraline and either MAO inhibitors, tryptophan or other drugs that elevate serotonin levels.

❑❑ What is the serotonin syndrome?

A toxic effect of some of the SSRIs or from using a SSRI along with a MAOI. It results from the combined effect of increasing serotonin stores plus inhibiting reuptake. Marked increases in serotonin in the synapses occur leading to a syndrome of hyperthermia, muscle rigidity, myoclonus and rapid changes in mental status and vital signs.

❑❑ What drugs are considered new generation antidepressants or newer atypical antidepressants?

Buproprion, mirtazapine, nefazodone and venlafaxine

❑❑ What is the mechanism of action of these newer atypical antidepressants?

They work on several neurotransmitter mechanisms, either through inhibition of reuptake or through direct receptor effects. They act differently from the other antidepressants.

❑❑ What are these atypical antidepressants used for?

They are used to treat major depressive disorders. In addition, venlafaxine has recently received an indication for the treatment of generalized anxiety disorder.

❑❑ What is the mechanism of action of bupropion?

It produces strong norepinephrine and significant dopamine reuptake inhibition.

❑❑ What is the advantage of using bupropion to treat depression?

It has a low incidence of anticholinergic effects and effects on sexual dysfunction and it actually causes weight loss.

❑❑ What is the principal disadvantage of bupropion?

It has amphetamine-like effects and is contraindicated in patients with seizure disorders.

❑❑ What are the adverse effects of bupropion?

Dizziness, dry mouth, sweating, tremor, aggravation of psychosis, and has a potential for seizures at high doses.

❑❑ What are the advantages of using nafazodone?

It has a low incidence of producing sexual dysfunction and a low incidence of cardiotoxicity.

❑❑ What are the adverse effects of nafazodone?

Drowsiness, dizziness, insomnia, nausea and agitation.

❑❑ What is the mechanism of action of mirtazapine?

It is an α_2-adrenergic receptor antagonist with potent $5HT_2$, $5HT_3$ and H_1 antagonist properties.

❑❑ What are the adverse effects of mirtazapine?

Most of the adverse effects are H1 receptor related and include sedation and weight gain.

❑❑ What herbal product has been claimed to be an effective antidepressant?

St Johns wort.

❑❑ What are the symptoms of mania?

The classic triad of manic symptoms consists of euphoria, psychomotor excitement and flight of ideas. Manic patients are considered "high" and are outgoing, overly alert, extravagant, and overly self confidant.

❑❑ What agents are used in the treatment of mania?

Lithium salts, carbamazepine and other agents such as valproic acid and clozapine.

❑❑ Which is the preferred drug for the treatment of mania?

Lithium carbonate.

❑❑ What is the main clinical use of lithium?

It is a mood stabilizing drug to prevent mood swings in patients with bipolar affective (manic-depressive) disorder. Because lithium has a slow onset of action concurrent use of antipsychotics may be required.

❑❑ What is the mechanism of action of lithium?

It exerts multiple biochemical effects but the exact mechanism is not known. It may effect electrolyte or ion transport, have effects on neurotransmitters, and have effects on second messengers. Its best known effect is on neurotransmitter signal transduction mechanisms. It causes G protein inhibition decreasing the inositol phosphate signaling pathway.

❑❑ Describe the pharmacokinetics of lithium?

It is well absorbed when given orally. There is a good correlation between the serum concentration and the therapeutic effect. Primarily the kidney eliminates it.

❑❑ What agents affect the plasma concentration of lithium?

Primarily sodium and water intake. The excretion of lithium absolutely depends on sodium.

❑❑ What are the adverse effects associated with lithium therapy?

Lithium has a low therapeutic index. Careful dosage adjustment and frequent monitoring of blood levels is necessary. Tremor is a frequent effect, GI upset, hypothyroidism, nephrogenic diabetes insipidus, edema and bradycardia-tachycardia (sick sinus) syndrome all can occur.

❒❒ What are the major drug interactions of lithium?

The combined use of iodine and lithium produces synergistic antithyroid effects, NSAIDS and the thiazide diuretics increase plasma lithium concentrations and antidepressants may precipitate mania.

DRUGS USED TO TREAT MIGRAINE

❒❒ How is serotonin synthesized?

It is synthesized from tryptophan in a reaction catalyzed by aromatic amino acid decarboxylase.

❒❒ Where is serotonin stored?

It is stored in synaptic vesicles in serotonergic neurons, platelets and enterochromaffin cells.

❒❒ What pharmacological actions does serotonin have?

It has many actions like histamine and has many species differences making generalizations difficult. Serotonin directly causes contraction of smooth muscle including GI smooth muscle. It has a small direct stimulant effect on bronchiolar smooth muscle in normal humans. It is potent stimulant of pain and itch sensory nerve endings and is responsible for some of the symptoms caused by insect and plant stings. It can mediate through a reflex bradycardia and hypotension. It participates in the vomiting reflex. It is a neurotransmitter in the brain and is also a precursor of melatonin.

❒❒ What is the mechanism of action of serotonin?

It acts through a variety of cell membrane receptors. Seven major subtypes have been identified. Six of these are G protein coupled and one is a ligand gated ion channel.

❒❒ Are serotonin and serotonin agonists useful clinically?

Serotonin itself has no clinical applications but several receptor subtype selective agonists are of clinical value. Buspirone is an anxiolytic. Dexfenfluramine is widely used as an appetite suppressant and sumatriptan is a $5HT_{1D}$ agonist effective in the treatment of migraine. Cisapride a $5HT_4$ agonist is used in the treatment of gastroesophageal reflux.

❒❒ How is serotonin metabolized?

There is a transporter for reuptake and it is metabolized by monamine oxidase and aldehyde dehydrogenase.

❒❒ What serotonin receptors are believed to be most important for the treatment of migraine?

$5HT_{1B}$ and $5HT_{1D}$

❒❒ What is migraine?

Migraine is a primary headache disorder. There is a steady or throbbing headache, which is most severe in the temporal or frontal regions. It is usually unilateral and is typically associated with nausea, vomiting, photophobia, phonophobia, and irritability.

❒❒ What is the pathophysiology of migraine headache?

Some vasomotor mechanism is involved. There is vasodilation of cranial blood vessels and plasma extravasation from cranial blood vessels. The aura is associated with an abnormal release of serotonin from the platelets while the throbbing headache is associated with decrease of platelet and serum serotonin below normal. There is also other evidence implicating serotonin in migraine.

❒❒ How is migraine headache diagnosed?

It must consist of any two of the following four features. Headache-unilateral site; headache-pulsating quality; associated nausea and associated photophobia or phonophobia.

❒❒ What are the general principles of pharmacotherapy for migraine headache?

Any drug will benefit no more than 60-70% of patients and you should begin acute therapy as soon as possible.

❒❒ Describe the therapy for mild, moderate and severe migraine?

Treatment generally follows the severity of the headache. For mild migraine you can use mild analgesics and antiemetics. For moderate migraine use a combination of analgesics, ergot alkaloids or triptans and antiemetics. For severe migraine use the ergot alkaloids, prophylactic treatment and antiemetics.

❒❒ What are the important pharmacological effects of the ergot alkaloids?

They cause vasoconstriction of most blood vessels and prevention of plasma extravasation. They also have a stimulant effect on the uterus. They have no significant effect on bronchiolar smooth muscle. Through an action of the GI tract they can produce nausea, vomiting and diarrhea.

❒❒ What is the mechanism of action of the ergot alkaloids?

They can act on several types of receptors including alpha adrenergic, dopamine and serotonin receptors. Their most important effect is stimulation of serotonin $5HT_{1B}$ and $5HT_{1D}$ receptors.

❏❏ **What is the main therapeutic use of the ergot alkaloids?**

Prevention and treatment of migraine.

❏❏ **How is ergotamine administered?**

It is available for all routes of administration, orally, sublingually, rectally, and IV, IM and by nasal spray.

❏❏ **How is dihydroergotamine administered?**

It is equally effective when given IV, IM, SC and nasally.

❏❏ **What are the adverse effects of the ergotamines?**

The most common adverse effects are GI disturbances including diarrhea, nausea, and vomiting. A more dangerous toxic effect of overdosage with agents like ergotamine and ergonovine is prolonged vasospasm. Other toxic effects include drowsiness.

❏❏ **What are the contraindications of the ergotamines?**

Pregnancy, peripheral vascular disease, coronary heart disease, hypertension, impaired hepatic or renal function.

❏❏ **Name four triptans used to treat migraine?**

Sumatriptan, naratriptan, rizatriptan and zolmitriptan.

❏❏ **What is the mechanism of action of the triptans?**

They are $5HT_1$ receptor agonists, especially the B and D subtypes.

❏❏ **How are the triptans used clinically?**

For the relief of symptoms of migraine headache.

❏❏ **What is a disadvantage of the triptans for migraine treatment?**

Their duration of effect is often shorter than the duration of the headache. As a result, several doses may be required during a prolonged migraine attack.

❏❏ **What are the adverse effects of the triptans?**

Pain, stinging or burning at the injection site. Also heaviness or pressure in the head, a feeling of warmth, chest discomfort and an increase in blood pressure.

❏❏ **What are the contraindications of the triptans?**

Ischemic heart disease and Prinzmetal's or variant angina.

❑❑ How and why is butorphanol used in treating migraine?

It is a partial opioid agonist. It is used as a nasal spray and has proven useful in reducing the pain due to migraine.

❑❑ Does butrophanol have side effects?

It has opoid like side effects. Cases of abuse have begun to appear.

❑❑ What drugs are used prophylactically for migraine?

Beta receptor antagonists (e.g. propranolol, timolol, atenolol, metoprolol, and nadolol; amitriptyline; methysergide.

ETHANOL

❑❑ Where is ethanol absorbed from?

Ethanol is rapidly absorbed from the stomach, small intestine and colon. Most absorption occurs form the first foot or so of the small intestine. Vaporized ethanol can be absorbed through the lungs.

❑❑ What enzyme is responsible for most of the metabolism of ethanol?

Alchohol dehydrogenase.

❑❑ What is the rate limiting factor in the metabolism of ethanol?

The rate of oxidation is relatively constant with time and is little increased by raising the blood concentration. The availability of NAD is rate limiting.

❑❑ What is acetaldehyde further metabolized too?

Acetic acid.

❑❑ What is the significance of the microsomal ethanol oxidizing system (MEOS)(Cytochrome P450 IIE1) in the metabolism of ethanol?

Ordinarily it plays a small role but chronic consumption of ethanol induces it and it may account for the increased rate of ethanol metabolism associated with chronic ethanol consumption.

❑❑ What effect does ethanol have on cytochrome P450 enzymes?

It induces some of these enzymes and inhibits others.

❑❑ From where is ethanol excreted?

Ethanol is excreted from all body fluids and in the breath.

❑❑ **Describe the mechanism of action of ethanol?**

It most likely acts at multiple sites including voltage gated ion channels, some calcium channels, and ligand gated ion channels. It also effects G-protein coupled receptors, inhibits some signal transduction pathways and has general membrane depressing effects.

❑❑ **What areas of the brain are depressed by ethanol?**

The most important areas depressed are the respiratory center, the thermoregulatory center and the pain centers.

❑❑ **How does ethanol interact with other CNS depressants?**

Ethanol has an additive effect with the other CNS depressants.

❑❑ **How does ethanol affect the cardiovascular system.**

It produces vasodilatation, a reduced incidence of coronary artery disease, an increase in HDL levels, and a decrease in platelet aggregation. Heavy drinkers may have hypertension, cardiac arrhythmias and cardiomyopathy. Some of the effects of ethanol are due to acetaldehyde.

❑❑ **What are the effects of the acetaldehyde that are produced by ethanol?**

Lipid peroxidation, damage to mitochondria and cellular enzymes, depletion of glutathione, vitamins and trace minerals.

❑❑ **What effects does ethanol have on metabolic systems of the body?**

Hyperglycemia, hypoglycemia, fatty acid deposits in the liver, and metabolic acidosis may occur.

❑❑ **What risks are associated with chronic consumption of ethanol?**

Alcoholism, cardiomyopathy, cirrhosis of the liver, gastritis, and neurological disorders.

❑❑ **What is the fetal alcohol syndrome?**

A syndrome describing the teratogenic effect of alcohol. The abnormality consists of CNS dysfunction, slowness in growth, a characteristic cluster of facial abnormalities and a variabl eset of major and minor malformations. These features may be in part due to a direct inhibitory effect of ethanol or acetaldehyde on embryonic cellular proliferation. Even moderate drinking is contraindicated during pregnancy.

❑❑ **What is the legal definition of ethanol intoxication?**

0.08-0.1% alcohol in the blood is prima facie evidence of being under the influence of alcohol. 0.05-0.1% is indicative of possibly being under the influence.

❑❑ **What are the primary goals of treating alcohol intoxication?**

Preventing the consequences of severe respiratory depression and aspiration of vomitus. Survival chances are good if the respiratory and cardiovascular systems are supported.

❑❑ What are the characteristics of alcohol withdrawal?

Minor symptoms include tremors, autonomic and somatic hyperactivity, insomnia mild confusion, irritability and agitation. Among the major symptoms are hallucinations and convulsions. With severe withdrawal there may be delirium tremens and arrhythmias.

❑❑ What are the DTs?

Delirium tremens which consists of tremor, anxiety, tachycardia, delusions and agitation. Chronic users of alcohol who suddenly stop taking it experience these.

❑❑ How is ethanol withdrawal treated?

The major objective of treating alcohol withdrawal is to prevent the development of seizures, delirium and arrhythmias. Benzodiazepines and clonidine are also useful.

❑❑ What is disulfiram used for?

Disulfiram is used to make alcohol consumption very undesirable. If alcohol is consumed after the person takes the disulfiram the patient becomes very sick.

❑❑ How does disulfiram work?

It inhibits acetaldehyde dehydrogenase, which results in the buildup of acetaldehyde.

❑❑ What are the consequences of consuming ethanol after having taken disulfiram?

There is intense flushing of the face and neck, an increased heart rate, dyspnea and hyperventilation, nausea and copious vomiting, decreased blood pressure and collapse and coma.

❑❑ Which drugs are widely known to cause a disulfiram type of reaction when taken along with ethanol?

Metronidazole, certain cephalosporins and the anticancer agent procarbazine.

❑❑ Why is naltrexone used in chronic ethanol abuse?

It decreases craving, decreases the number of days in which alcohol is consumed and decreases the incidence of binge drinking.

❑❑ What are some of the widely accepted uses of ethanol?

It is used topically as a cleansing agent It is also used to deaden nerves producing chronic pain and to treat methanol and ethylene glycol poisoning.

❑❑ What types of drug interactions are characteristic of ethanol?

It can inhibit and induce certain microsomal enzymes and thus can affect drugs metabolized by those systems. It can increase the bleeding caused by salicylates and other NSAIDS. It can produce additive orthostatic hypotension when used with other vasodilators. With insulin and the oral hypoglycemic agents it can produce severe hypoglycemia and it interferes with the metabolism of oral hypoglycemics. If given with MAO inhibitors you can get a hypertensive crisis due to the tyramine present in certain foods and drinks.

MUSCLE RELAXANTS

❑❑ What are the different types of drugs used as muscle relaxants?

There are centrally acting drugs used to treat muscle spasticity and drugs used to treat muscle spasms and there are drugs which act locally to block the muscle contraction that produces muscle spasticity and neuromuscular blocking agents that produce total muscle paralysis.

❑❑ What is meant by muscle spasticity?

It stems from injury to nerve cells at any of the various centers in the cerebrospinal axis that contribute to the control of muscle tone and to the coordination of complex movements. In spasticity there is an imbalance in the regulation of the motor nerve causing the muscle fiber to respond to stretch in an exaggerated manner.

❑❑ What drugs are used to treat muscle spasticity?

Centrally acting drugs like diazepam and baclofen and drugs that act directly on the muscle like dantrolene sodium.

❑❑ What is the mechanism by which diazepam decreases muscle spasticity?

It decreases the release of the excitatory neurotransmitter from primary afferent nerve endings probably by acting on the $GABA_A$ receptor Cl^- channel complex.

❑❑ How does baclofen act to decrease muscle spasticity?

It acts as an agonist at the $GABA_B$ receptor located on the primary afferent nerve ending in the spinal cord. These receptors block the release of the excitatory nerurotransmitter possibly by blocking Ca^{++} channels in the nerve ending.

❑❑ How is diazepam used clinically in spasticity?

It is used to decrease spasticity especially in patients with lesions affecting the spinal cord and occasionally in patients with cerebral palsy. It is not particularly helpful for spasticity caused by strokes. It is not effective in rigidity associated with parkinsonism or huntington's disease.

❑❑ What are the adverse effects associated with diazepam use to decrease spasticity?

Sedation is most common. Impaired coordination, weakness, dizziness, mental confusion and ataxia also may occur and addiction and physical dependence may occur on chronic usage.

❑❑ What is the principal use of baclofen?

To decrease spasticity caused by multiple sclerosis and spinal cord injury. It also decreases the pain associated with spasticity. It is not recommended in patients following strokes or other cerebral lesions.

❑❑ What are the most common side effects associated with the use of baclofen?

Drowsiness, insomnia, dizziness, weakness, ataxia and mental confusion and GI distress. Sudden withdrawal after chronic use may result in auditory and visual hallucinations, anxiety, tachycardia and a rebound increase in the number of flexor spasms. At toxic doses it can cause coma, respiratory depression and seizures.

❑❑ What is the mechanism of action of dantrolene?

It reduces the depolarization-induced release of calcium from the sarcoplasmic reticulum and thus blocks muscle contraction.

❑❑ What are the main uses of dantrolene?

Dantrolene is used to decrease spasticity, in patients with upper motor neuron lesions. It is especially useful in patients whose nursing care is made difficult by severe, prolonged muscle contraction and who will not be troubled by any concomitant decrease in voluntary power. It is effective for patients with strokes and spinal cord injury. It is also used to prevent and/or treat malignant hyperthermia and the neuroleptic malignant syndrome.

❑❑ What is malignant hypothermia?

An autosomal dominant trait that is triggered by certain drugs such as general anesthetics or succinylcholine. There is rapid metabolism in muscle along with rigor and destruction of muscle tissue.

❑❑ What are the adverse reactions associated with dantrolene use?

The most serious effect is hepatotoxicity. Drowsiness, dizziness, general malaise, fatigues and diarrhea are frequent and muscle weakness is common.

❑❑ What causes muscle spasms?

They are caused by injury to the muscle rather than the nerve. For example, over stretching a muscle, wrenching a joint, or tearing tendons or ligament can cause violent involuntary muscle contractions. There is an excessive stream of sensory impulses that pass to the nervous system from the injured part.

❑❑ Name five drugs used for the treatment of muscle spasms?

Carisoprodol, chlorphenesin, chlorzoxazone, cyclobenzaprine, diazepam, methocarbamol, orphenadrine and several NSAIDS.

❑❑ What is the mechanism of action of the drugs used to treat muscle spasms?

They depress spinal polysynaptic reflexes preferentially over monosynaptic reflexes as well as facilitative and inhibitory neuronal activity affecting muscle stretch reflexes.

❑❑ What adverse effects do all of these drugs treating muscle spasms have in common?

Drowsiness is common to most of them.

❑❑ What precautions apply to all spasmolytics?

Patients receiving these drugs should not undertake activities that require mental alertness, judgment, and physical coordination. CNS depressant effect may be additive with other CNS depressants including alcohol. Physical and psychic dependence may develop after long-term use. Abrupt withdrawal may produce severe withdrawal symptoms including seizures.

NEUROMUSCULAR BLOCKING AGENTS

❑❑ What are the two groups of commonly used neuromuscular blocking agents

Nondepolarising or competitive blocking agents and the depolarizing agents.

❑❑ Give one or two examples of each of these groups used as neuromuscular blocking agents?

Tubocurarine and pancuronium are nondepolarizing agents while succinylcholine is a depolarizing agent.

❑❑ What is the mechanism of action of the competitive blockers?

They are antagonists at the nicotinic acetylcholine receptor in the neuromuscular junction. They bind to the acetylcholine receptor but do not open the ion channel and do not change the membrane potential at all.

❑❑ What effect does an acetylcholinesterase inhibitor have on a competitive block?

It results in a build up of acetylcholine and a reversal of the block. The excess acetylcholine competes with the competitive blocker and can reverse the effects of the competitive blocker.

❑❑ How does the depolarizing blocker succinylcholine work?

It is an agonist at the nicotinic receptor in the neuromuscular junction. The binding of succinylcholine causes the channel in the nicotinic receptor to open. Sodium rushes into the endplate, an endplate potential and muscle action potential occurs and the surrounding muscle contracts. There is persistent depolarization of the endplate preventing a new action potential from occurring. The surrounding muscle fiber relaxes as it reaches a state of accomodation and relaxes. In phase II block which occurs after a single large dose, repeated administration or prolonged infusion of succinylcholine the acetylcholine receptor becomes sensitized to the effects of succinylcholine but the muscle remains paralyzed.

❑❑ Compare the pattern of muscle contraction with competitive blocking agents vs. depolarizing agents if the ulnar nerve is stimulated with the muscle only partially paralyzed?

After a train of four with a competitive blocker you get a fade or decrease with each successive stimulation. With a depolarizing agent you get a constant but diminished pattern of contraction. After tetanic stimulation you get similar results. If there is pause after the tetanic stimulation and then the nerve is stimulated again, you get a contraction greater than the initial stimulation (posttetanic potentiation) with competitive blockers but not with depolarizing agents.

❑❑ Compare the duration of action of succinylcholine vs. the competitive blocking agents?

Succinylcholine has a very short duration due to diffusion of drug out of the neuromuscular junction to other tissues of the body. With the competitive agents duration is due to redistribution of the drug from the neuromuscular junction to other body tissues and is considerably longer than with succinylcholine.

❑❑ What are the adverse effects of succinylcholine?

In children given low doses of the drug there will be stimulation of muscarinic receptors in the heart and bradycardia. In adults with high doses you get stimulation of nicotinic receptors in the autonomic ganglia to produce cardiac arrhythmias and an increase in blood pressure.

❑❑ What are the adverse effects of tubocurarine?

The rapid IV injection of large doses of tubocurarine in humans may cause a rapid and severe fall in blood pressure. The major cause of this hypotension is peripheral vasodilatation resulting from the release of histamine and sympathetic ganglionic blockade.

❑❑ What are the adverse effects of pancuronium?

Its primary adverse effect is to block muscarinic receptors in the heart producing tachycardia and a slight rise in blood pressure.

❑❑ What are the drug-drug interactions associated with the use of the neuromuscular blocking agents?

Drugs, which decrease muscle contraction, will potentiate the effects of neuromuscular blocking agents. From a clinical viewpoint the most important pharmacological interactions of these drugs are with certain general anesthetics, some antibiotics and calcium channel blockers. Acetylcholinesterase inhibitors on the other hand reverse the action of the competitive blockers.

❑❑ What precautions and contraindications must be considered before using the neuromuscular blocking agents?

In diseases affecting muscle contraction such as amyotrophic latereral sclerosis and myasthenia gravis. In patients with burns or muscular denervations there is an increase in serum potassium levels following succinylcholine. Succinylcholine shouldn't be used in patients with atypical plasma cholinesterase and succinylcholine may precipitate a malignant hyperthermic crisis in genetically predisposed patients.

❑❑ What are the therapeutic uses of the neuromuscular blocking agents?

Their primary use is to produce muscle paralysis during surgical procedures. Minor uses include prevention of muscle contraction during electroshock therapy and using them to allow for artificial ventilation when a patient is unresponsive to antiepiletptic therapy.

❑❑ Do the neuromuscular blocking agents have any analgesic effect?

None.

LOCAL ANESTHETICS

❑❑ Describe the general properties of local anesthetics?

These are drugs injected near a nerve and act at the site of injection. They block the flow of electrons along the axon and consequently they block pain without loss of consciousness and their effects are reversible.

❑❑ Describe the general structural features of local anesthetics?

They contain a lipophilic group connected to a hydrophilic group through an intermediate chain. The intermediate linkage is either an ester or an amide.

❑❑ Which local anesthetics have an ester linkage?

Cocaine, procaine, benzocaine and tetracaine.

❑❑ Which local anesthetics have an amide linkage?

Lidocaine, bupivacaine and mepivacaine.

❑❑ What is the clinical significance of the type of intermediate linkage that is present in local anesthetics?

Most ester-linked drugs are metabolized in the plasma by plasma cholinesterase. The amide-linked drugs are metabolized in the liver.

❏❏ Hypersensitivity to local anesthetics occurs as a result of what portion of the drug?

It is due to the p-aminobenzoic acid (PABA) portion and its derivatives.

❏❏ What type of cross sensitivity occurs with the local anesthetics?

It occurs between benzoic acid and PABA. It does not occur between esters and amides or between aniline and quinoline derivatives.

❏❏ What is the mechanism of action of the local anesthetics?

The primary mechanism of action is blockade of voltage gated sodium channels. They appear to diffuse into the sodium channel when the channel is in the open state. They subsequently block the channel and increase the amount of energy required to convert the channel back to the resting state.

❏❏ What factors determine the minimal concentration of a local anesthetic required to block nerve transmission?

The potency of the anesthetic, the site of injection in comparison to the location of the nerve, the pKa of the drug, the pH of the tissue surrounding the nerve membrane, the diameter of the nerve fiber and the rate at which the nerve is firing.

❏❏ How does pH effect the action of local anesthetics?

Local anesthetics are generally marketed as water-soluble salts usually hydrochlorides. Inasmuch as the local anesthetics are weak bases their hydrochloride salts are mildly acidic. This property increases the stability of the local anesthetic esters and any accompanying vasoconstrictor substance. Although the unprotonated form is necessary for diffusion across cellular membranes, the cationic form interacts preferentially with sodium channels. Altering the pH can block the action of the local anesthetics.

❏❏ Describe the order in which sensory nerve function is blocked by local anesthetics?

Pain, temperature, touch, deep pressure, and motor nerves.

❏❏ What is the order of recovery of nerves blocked by local anesthetics?

It is the reverse order from blockage with pain returning last.

❏❏ The absorption of a local anesthetic from the site of injection depends on what factors?

The most important factor is the blood supply at the injection site. The greater the blood supply the faster the rate of absorption. Areas of high blood supply include the trachea, bronchi and floor of the mouth.

❑❑ The rate of onset of the local anesthetics is controlled by what factors?

The dosage of the drug given and how close to the nerve you give the drug.

❑❑ What factors control the duration of action of the local anesthetics?

The duration is proportional to the time during which the anesthetic is in contact with the nerve. Procedures that keep the drug at the nerve prolong the duration time. The rate of absorption into the blood stream also is important.

❑❑ What drug is used to reduce the rate of uptake of local anesthetics?

Epinephrine.

❑❑ What is the mechanism by which epinephrine reduces local anesthetic uptake?

Vasoconstriction.

❑❑ What is the recommended concentration of epinephrine for reducing local anesthetic uptake?

1:200,000

❑❑ What are some of the adverse effects of the local anesthetics?

Inhibition of muscle contraction, vasodilation at the injection site (except cocaine), and bradycardia.

❑❑ Why does cocaine cause vasoconstriction rather than vasodilation?

It inhibits the reuptake of norepinephrine into the nerve ending.

❑❑ What are the toxic effects of the local anesthetics on the CNS?

Following absorption local anesthetics may cause stimulation of the CNS producing restlessness and tremor that may progress to convulsions. Central stimulation is followed by depression. You may see stimulation only, stimulation followed by depression or depression only. There is stimulation of the cerebral cortex with light-headedness, visual and auditory disturbances, tinnitus, excitement, disorientation, incoherent speech and convulsions. With depression there is unconsciousness, depression of the respiration and decreases in blood pressure and heart rate.

❑❑ How are the toxic effects of the local anesthetics treated?

You should maintain an airway, support respiration and treat the cardiovascular symptoms.

❑❑ What types of hypersensitivity reactions occur with the local anesthetics?

These are uncommon but may consist of allergic dermatitis, a typical asthmatic attack and possibly fatal anaphylactic reactions.

❑❑ What substance may be causing the allergic reactions associated with the local anesthetics?

The preservative methylparaben.

❑❑ What are the clinical uses of the local anesthetics?

Infiltration anesthesia, topical anesthesia, field block anesthesia, nerve block anesthesia, IV regional anesthesia, spinal anesthesia and epidural anesthesia.

GENERAL ANESTHETICS

❑❑ What is meant by the term anesthetic state?

The anesthetic state is a drug-induced state that makes the subject amnestic and relatively unresponsive to painful stimuli.

❑❑ What kinds of drugs are used to obtain the anesthetic state?

General inhalation anesthetics (gases and volatile liquids) and IV anesthetics which are used mainly to induce anesthesia.

❑❑ What are the desirable physiological characteristics for a patient during surgical procedures?

There should be amnesia and unconsciousness. The patient should be unresponsive to painful stimuli. There should be cardiovascular stability and the muscles should be relaxed to facilitate intubation. The level of CNS depression should be controllable.

❑❑ What IV anesthetics are used to obtain the anesthetic state?

Thiopental, propofol, droperidol, fentanyl and ketamine. Some of these are used to induce anesthesia and some to produce general anesthesia.

❑❑ How is thiopental used clinically?

It is used to induce anesthesia in combination with inhaled anesthetics.

❑❑ What accounts for the fast onset of action of thiopental as well as its short duration?

It has high lipid solubility and thus crosses the blood-brain barrier very quickly. It quickly diffuses out of the brain and other highly vascularized organs and is rapidly redistributed to muscle, fat and other body tissues, which accounts for its short duration.

❑❑ What side effects does thiopental have?

It may induce laryngospasm and bronchospasm. It may also exacerbate acute intermittent porphyria.

❒❒ What are the therapeutic uses of the diazepams in anesthesia?

They are used for preoperative sedation, intraoperative sedation for procedures not requiring analgesia and as part of balanced anesthesia.

❒❒ Why is midazolam used as a pre-anesthetic medication?

It produces antegrade anmesia and calms the patient.

❒❒ What adverse effects are associated with the use of benzodiazepines in anesthesia?

Alone they cause moderate circulatory and respiratory depression. If used with opioids cardiovascular collapse and respiratory arrest can occur.

❒❒ What are the uses for propofol?

It is used to induce anesthesia.

❒❒ Why is propofol preferred over thiopental for induction of anesthesia?

The recovery is quicker and the patients are able to get up sooner than with other IV anesthetics. There are less nausea and emesis and no cumulative effect from propofol administration or delayed recovery after prolonged infusion.

❒❒ What is meant by balanced anesthesia?

Using an inductive agent, an opioid analgesic, a neuromuscular blocking agent and nitrous oxide together.

❒❒ What types of supplemental drugs are used during general anesthesia?

Benzodiazepines are used to calm the patient and decrease the amount of anesthetic needed, analgesics such as fentanyl, neuromuscular blocking agents, agents used to maintain the cardiovascular system (mainly atropine), and agents used to prevent salivary secretion (mainly glycopyrrolate).

❒❒ Why is midazolam preferred to diazepam as the benzodiazepine of choice during anesthesia?

It has a rapid onset, shorter duration and produces a lower incidence of thrombophlebitis.

❒❒ What is the mechanism of action of the general anesthetics?

Most likely their action results from an action directly on proteins. Anesthetics appear to alter the ability of proteins to change conformation by acting directly on the protein and/or by altering the fluidity of the membrane and /or the hydrophobicity of the environment surrounding the protein. Ligand gated ion channels have been found to be particularly sensitive to general anesthetics but G protein linked receptors and some voltage gated calcium channels are affected.

❑❑ What is the Meyer-Overton theory of general anesthetics?

It refers to the close correlation of anesthetic potency with lipid solubility.

❑❑ Is there an anesthetic receptor?

There doesn't seem to be a specific anesthetic receptor.

❑❑ What are the phases of administration of the general anesthetics?

Induction, maintenance and emergence.

❑❑ What are the advantages and disadvantages of general anesthetics compared to intravenous anesthetics?

With the general anesthetics the anesthesiologist has ready control over the depth of anesthesia. If CNS depression gets too high, the concentration of anesthetic in the inspired mixture can be decreased and CNS depression can be readily reversed. The patient can be titrated with anesthetic and you are not dependent on metabolism or excretion to eliminate the drug from the body. With IV anesthetics you get a very rapid action and increased CNS depression can be readily achieved by giving more drug. If CNS depression is too high it is difficult to reverse a toxic dose as metabolism and excretion are required to eliminate the drug from the body.

❑❑ Define induction of anesthesia?

The time from administration of a general anesthetic to the achievement of surgical anesthesia.

❑❑ What is the induction of anesthesia dependent on?

How fast the anesthetic reaches the CNS.

❑❑ What factors affect the rate of induction of an anesthetic?

The solubility of the anesthetic, the degree of pulmonary ventilation, the partial pressure of the inhaled agent, the alveolar blood flow and the arteriovenous concentration gradient.

❑❑ How does solubility of the anesthetic agent affect the rate of induction?

The more aqueous soluble the inhalation anesthetic agent the longer the time required for induction (the slower the induction).

❑❑ How does the rate of pulmonary ventilation affect the induction rate?

For an aqueous soluble agent an increased rate of respiration speeds up the rate of induction.

❑❑ How does partial pressure of the inhaled agent affect the induction rate?

An increased concentration in the inhaled air leads to a greater concentration at the alveoli and thus increases the arterial partial pressure of the agent. This will speed up induction.

❑❑ How does alveolar blood flow affect the induction rate?

An increased blood flow allows for more rapid uptake of the agent and quicker effect on the CNS.

❑❑ How does the arteriovenous concentration gradient affect the induction rate?

A high rate and extent of tissue uptake will decrease the venous concentration of an anesthetic. As a result it will take a longer time for the anesthetic concentration of arterial and venous blood to equilibrate.

❑❑ What factors are important in determining the duration of action of the general anesthetics?

The major factor involved is redistribution from the brain to other body tissues.

❑❑ Define emergence (recovery)?

Emergence is the reverse of induction. It is the time from the discontinuance of the anesthetic until the patient awakens and breathes on his own.

❑❑ What does emergence from anesthesia depend on?

How quickly the anesthetic is removed from the CNS.

❑❑ What signs indicate the tension of an anesthetic agent is too low?

The tension is too low when there are tears, swallowing, increased resistance to inflation of the lungs, irregular breathing, increased heart rate and blood pressure and apnea following peritoneal stimulation.

❑❑ How is the potency of general anesthetics measured?

At a given level of anesthesia the measurement of the steady state alveolar concentrations of different anesthetics provides a comparison of their relative potencies. By measuring the MAC you can determine the potency.

❑❑ What is meant by MAC?

It is the minimal alveolar concentration of an anesthetic that will prevent muscular movements upon painful stimulation in 50% of the total subjects.

❑❑ How does MAC relate to potency?

The greater the MAC of an anesthetic, the greater the concentration needed to provide anesthesia. Thus an agent with a high MAC has a low potency.

❑❑ What factors affect the amount of inhalation anesthetic agents required producing anesthesia?

Anesthesia depends on the tension of the anesthetic present in the neuronal membrane. This in turn depends on the solubility of the drug in the highly lipid nerve membranes compared to its solubility in blood and in the cytosol.

❑❑ What factors affect the distribution of the general anesthetics?

The volume of the tissue compartment, the lipid content of the tissue, the difference in tension between the tissue and blood and the solubility of gas in the blood vs. the tissue.

❑❑ What is meant by the term concentration effect?

When higher concentrations of an anesthetic gas are inhaled the arterial tension increases at a greater rate than it would have if a lesser concentration of the anesthetic had been inhaled. When an inhalation agent is given in high tension a large volume of gas may pass through the lung and enter the blood in a short time. This creates negative pressure in the lung, which causes more gas to flow into the lung.

❑❑ What is meant by the term second gas effect?

When two gases are administered simultaneously one in high tension and the other in low tension, the negative pressure created by uptake of the gas administered in high tension causes more of both gases to be taken into the lung.

❑❑ How does the emergence time compare to the induction time?

The two times are about the same.

❑❑ What is meant by diffusion hypoxia?

It is the reverse of the concentration effect? The presence of a gas dilutes the available oxygen in the alveoli and thus reduces the concentration of oxygen. It is seen following the administration of nitrous oxide if the patient is breathing air. Administering oxygen for the first few minutes after you stop the nitrous oxide can prevent it.

❑❑ What are the major physical properties of nitrous oxide?

It is a non-explosive, non-flammable gas. It is the least lipid soluble and least aqueous soluble of the anesthetics.

❑❑ Is nitrous oxide a good analgesic?

Yes, 20-35 vol% is equal to about 10 mg morphine.

❑❑ How is nitrous oxide used clinically?

It is used for the induction of general anesthesia but is not used as the sole anesthetic because of the danger of hypoxia.

❑❑ How is nitrous oxide administered?

It is inhaled but must be used in conjunction with other anesthetics because of its low potency.

❑❑ Is nitrous oxide a good muscle relaxant?

No, it is a poor muscle relaxant.

❑❑ What are the toxic effects of nitrous oxide?

It can cause bone marrow depression with prolonged administration. High concentrations can cause neuropathies, but it has very little effect on the respiratory and cardiovascular systems.

❑❑ What special considerations should be taken into account during the recovery phase when using nitrous oxide?

Care must be taken to adequately oxygenate the patient otherwise diffusion hypoxia may occur.

❑❑ What are the major physical and chemical properties of halothane?

It is a halogenated hydrocarbon. It is a volatile liquid but it is non-flammable and non-explosive. It is a very lipid soluble agent and also one of the more aqueous soluble anesthetics.

❑❑ What are the clinical indications for halothane?

Its use as a general anesthetic has declined in recent years because of the possibility of hepatitis and the availability of safer agents.

❑❑ Describe the effects of halothane on the heart?

Halothane has dose dependent effects on the cardiovascular system. Halothane sensitizes the myocardium to the effects of catecholamines (thus increasing the risk of arrhythmia), it decreases the heart rate and cardiac output, and leads to lowered blood pressure and peripheral resistance.

❑❑ What are the advantages of combining nitrous oxide with halothane?

The combination decreases the amount of halothane needed, reduces CNS depression and decreases adverse cardiovascular effects. The combination also increases the analgesic effects and speeds up the rate of induction through a second gas effect.

❑❑ What is the mechanism of the hepatitis associated with halothane use?

As a result of metabolism chemically reactive or immunogenic products may be formed. A large amount of these toxic products may be a primary factor in production of hepatitis.

❏❏ What other toxic effects have been associated with halothane use?

Malignant hyperthermia.

❏❏ Describe the physical properties of isoflurane?

It is less aqueous soluble and less lipid soluble than halothane. Its use allows a faster induction and recovery than with halothane.

❏❏ What are the advantages and disadvantages of isoflurane?

It has a more pungent odor than halothane and supplemental IV agents are used to overcome this disadvantage. Anesthesia with isoflurane is associated with progressive respiratory depression and hypotension. Like halothane it has the potential for malignant hyperthermia. It does not sensitize the myocardium to catecholamines and does not induce arrhythmia and the depth of anesthesia can be adjusted rapidly.

❏❏ What are the advantages and disadvantages of sevoflurane?

Blood pressure decreases to the same extent, as with other inhalation anesthetics, tachycardia is not as likely as with isoflurane and it does not sensitize the heart to circulating catecholamines. There is more respiratory depression than with halothane and it is not as irritating to the respiratory tract as isoflurane. Hepatitis has not been reported after sevofluarane.

CARDIOVASCULAR/PULMONARY PHARMACOLOGY

ANTIASTHMATICS

❑❑ Asthma is now considered to be mainly what type of disease?

Inflammatory.

❑❑ What are the clinical symptoms of asthma?

Shortness of breath, coughing, wheezing and chest tightness.

❑❑ What triggers an asthmatic attack?

Various allergens, infections (e.g. viral) and psychological factors.

❑❑ What is the mechanism of action of epinephrine when used to treat asthma?

It is a nonselective beta agonist, causing bronchodilation.

❑❑ How is epinephrine used in the treatment of asthma?

It is used as an inhalant for its short acting effects and given subcutaneously for acute asthmatic attacks.

❑❑ Name two selective beta agonists used in the treatment of asthma?

Albuterol, terbutaline, bitolterol and pirbuterol

❑❑ What is the mechanism of action of albuterol (as well as terbutaline, bitolterol etc.) in the treatment of asthma?

They are selective beta agonists consequently they produce bronchodilation.

❑❑ How are these beta agonists usually administered?

They are usually inhaled but also can be given orally.

❑❑ How are they used clinically in the treatment of asthma?

They are used to treat acute bronchospasm and exercise induced asthma.

❑❑ What side effects are usually associated with the use of the beta agonists?

Tachycardia, palpitations and tremor and at high doses hypokalemia.

❑❑ What advantage is there to using oral preparations of beta agonists?

They are useful in some young children with mild symptoms who can't use an inhaler and spacer device.

❑❑ What is salmeterol?

A long acting $beta_2$ selective agonist.

❑❑ What is salmeterol used for clinically?

In the treatment of asthma, for maintenance therapy and in patients with nocturnal symptoms.

❑❑ What can the long term daily use of salmeterol lead to ?

Tolerance.

❑❑ What is ipratropium?

It is an atropine derivative.

❑❑ What is the mechanism of action of ipratropium?

It competitively inhibits muscarinic receptors and blocks vagal stimulated bronchoconstriction.

❑❑ How is ipratropium used therapeutically?

It is used in the treatment of asthma. It is given in an inhaler and is very useful in the elderly and in combination with a $beta_2$ agonist for acute severe asthma. It is also used to treat chronic obstructive pulmonary disease.

❑❑ What are the adverse effects of ipratropium?

Dry mouth and pharyngeal irritation and it may increase intraocular pressure in glaucoma patients.

❑❑ Why is theophylline useful in asthma?

It is a bronchodilator.

❑❑ What is the mechanism of action of theophylline?

The exact mechanism is unknown. It has been hypothesized that it may inhibit adenosine receptors, inhibit phosphodiesterase and act as an antiinflammatory agent.

❑❑ How is theophylline currently used for the treatment of asthma?

It is used for persistent asthma, especially nocturnal asthma. It has limited usefulness for acute asthma.

❑❑ What are the adverse effects of theophylline?

They depend on the plasma levels with few adverse effects occurring below 10 mg/ml. At concentrations higher than 20 mg/ml there is nausea, nervousness, anxiety, headache and insomnia. At concentrations above 40 mg/ml there is vomiting, hypocalcemia, hyperglycemia, tachycardia, cardiac arrhythmias, tremor, neuromuscular irritability and seizures.

❑❑ Are there many drug interactions involving theophylline?

This is another drawback of using theophylline. It interacts with many drugs and foods. Many of which increase or decrease theophylline's concentration. Among them, are cimetidine and erythromycin, phenytoin and quinolones.

❑❑ How do cromolyn and nedocromil work?

They are anti-inflammatory. They act mainly to prevent release of mediators from activated mast cells.

❑❑ How are cromolyn and nedocromil used in asthma treatment?

They are inhalants used strictly as prophylactics. They provide no relief from acute attacks.

❑❑ What are the adverse effects of cromolyn and nedocromil?

They have minimal adverse effects with some reflex wheezing. Nedocromil has a bad taste associated with its use.

❑❑ How do the steroids work to treat asthma?

They act through their antiinflammatory effects. They bind to glucocorticoid receptors and inhibit inflammation at multiple sites including reversing mucosal edema, decreasing capillary permeability and inhibiting the release of various cytokines.

❑❑ What type of steroid preparations are most commonly used to treat asthma?

The inhaled preparations are preferred as they have less toxicity.

❑❑ Name four steroids used as inhalants to treat asthma?

Budesonide, fluticasone, beclomethasone and flunisolide.

❑❑ How are the steroids used in the treatment of asthma?

They are used to treat mild to moderate persistent asthma as well as severe asthma.

❒❒ What toxicity is associated with the use of inhaled steroids?

Hoarseness and oral candidiasis can occur. Growth impairment in children, suppression of the hypothalamic-pituitary adrenal axis, decreased bone density, cataract formation and with high doses dermal thickening and glaucoma are possibilities also.

❒❒ What is the use for oral and parenteral steroids in the treatment of asthma?

For acute exacerbations of asthma unresponsive to bronchodilators.

❒❒ What types of toxicity are associated with the use of systemic steroids?

There are many and some are very serious. There may be weight gain, hypertension and adrenal suppression and changes in glucose metabolism.

❒❒ What is the rationale behind the use of leukotriene modifiers in the treatment of asthma?

Leukotrienes are recognized to have an important role in inflammation. They can cause eosinophil migration, mucus production and airway wall edema and bronchoconstriction. Antagonists block production of leukotrienes or act as receptor antagonists.

❒❒ What is zafirlukast?

A leukotriene receptor antagonist.

❒❒ How is zarfirlukast used clinically?

For asthma maintenance therapy.

❒❒ What are the side effects of zarfirlukast therapy?

Mild headache, GI disturbances, and elevated liver enzymes.

❒❒ What is the mechanism of action of zileuton?

It is a leukotriene synthesis inhibitor.

❒❒ How is zileuton used in the treatment of asthma?

For the maintenance treatment of asthma.

❒❒ What is status asthmaticus?

An asthmatic crisis. It is a life-threatening attack of asthma. A sudden intense and continuous aggravation of the asthmatic state.

❒❒ How is status asthmaticus treated?

With IV steroids and bronchodilators.

ANTIHISTAMINES

❑❑ Histamine receptors fall into which group of receptors?

G protein coupled receptors.

❑❑ How many subgroups of histamine receptors are there?

H_1, H_2, and H_3

❑❑ What agent is a physiological antagonist of histamine?

Epinephrine.

❑❑ What compounds serve as histamine release inhibitors?

Cromolyn, nedocromil and some $beta_2$ adrenergic agonists.

❑❑ What drugs are H_2 histamine receptor blockers?

Cimetidine, ranitidine, famotidine and nizatidine.

❑❑ Describe the major pharmacokinetic properties of the H_1 receptor blockers?

They are rapidly absorbed following oral administration, widely distributed throughout the body, extensively metabolized by the liver microsomal enzyme system and have a relatively short duration of action.

❑❑ What are the pharmacological properties of the H_1 histamine receptor blockers?

They inhibit most responses of smooth muscle to histamine, and block the action of histamine to increase permeability and formation of edema and wheal. They also stimulate and depress the CNS, and have anticholinergic, local anesthetic, antinausea and antiemetic, antiparkinson, adrenoreceptor blocking actions, and serotonin blocking effects.

❑❑ What are the major differences between the first and second-generation antihistamines?

The second generation compounds do not produce CNS sedation and anticholinergic effects.

❑❑ What are the common therapeutic uses for the H_1-specific antihistamines?

The major use is for seasonal allergic rhinitis and conjunctivitis. Other uses include urticaria, dermatitis, insect bites, poison ivy, motion sickness, vestibular disturbances and as local anesthetics.

❑❑ What are the major adverse effects of the H_1 histamine blockers?

Daytime drowsiness, CNS stimulation, appetite and GI disorders, dry mouth and sinuses., allergic reactions and arrhythmias.

❑❑ What is the major adverse effect associated with the second-generation H_1 histamine blockers?

Arrhythmias.

❑❑ What is the mechanism of the arrhythmias caused by the second generation H_1 histamine blockers?

The second-generation compounds which are prodrugs bind to cardiac K^+ channels and may cause polymorphic ventricular tachycardias ("torsades de point").

❑❑ What agents or situations may result in an increased likelihood of arryhythmias occurring from these drugs?

Liver dysfunction, ingestion of grapefruit juice, therapy with other drugs that are inhibitors of the CYP 450 3A4 isoenzyme, and an increased tendency towards arryhthymias.

❑❑ Why doesn't fexofenadine produce arrhythmias?

It is a metabolite of terfenadine rather than a prodrug.

ANTIARRHYTHMIC DRUGS

❑❑ What are cardiac arrhythmias?

Any rhythm that is not under the usual autonomic control or one that does not start at the SA node.

❑❑ What are the three basic origins of arrhythmias?

Abnormal automaticity, triggered activity, and reentry.

❑❑ What are the two types of cardiac tissue from an electrophysiological view and where are they located?

Fast response and slow response. Slow response tissue includes the SA and AV nodes and fast response tissue includes the Purkinje cells and in the myocardium.

❑❑ What are the different classes of antiarrhythmic drugs?

Class I -sodium channel blockers; Class II-β-adrenergic receptor blockers; Class III-potassium channel blockers; Class IV-calcium channel blockers. Several of these drugs have properties of more than one class.

❑❑ What are the effects of sodium channel blockers on the heart?

They slow the rate of phase 0 depolarization, reduce conduction velocity and elevate the excitability threshold and increase the QRS complex duration.

❑❑ What are the effects of potassium channel blockers on the heart?

They delay repolarization, prolong action potential duration, prolong the refractory period and increase the QT interval.

❑❑ What effects do calcium channel blockers have on the heart?

In slow tissue they reduce the rate of phase 0 depolarization, reduce conduction velocity, reduce excitability and increase the P-R interval.

❑❑ What is the mechanism of action of the class I_A drugs?

They have moderate phase 0 depression, slow conduction velocity and prolong repolarization (K^+ blocking effect).

❑❑ Name the class I_A antiarrhythmic drugs?

Quinidine, procainamide and disopyramide.

❑❑ What is the mechanism of action of quinidine?

To a large extent the actions of quinidine result from its ability to block activated sodium channels. Recovery from the block is slower and less complete in depolarized than in fully polarized tissue. Thus, quinidine lengthens the refractory period and depresses excitability and conduction in depolarized tissue more than in normal tissue.

❑❑ What therapeutic uses do the class Ia drugs have?

They are secondary drugs for supraventricular and ventricular arrhythmias.

❑❑ How is quinidine given?

Orally.

❑❑ How is procainamide given?

Orally, IV or IM.

❑❑ What is the major metabolite of procainamide?

N-acetylprocainamide (NAPA) which is proarrhythmic.

❑❑ What are the major toxicities of quinidine on the heart?

SA block, torsade de pointes, paradoxical increases in ventricular rates when given for atrial flutter/fibrillatiion, asystole or arrhythmias if the QRS complex is wider.

❑❑ What are the non-cardiac adverse effects of quinidine?

Cinchonism, GI disturbances, and hypotension.

❑❑ If digoxin and quinidine are given concurrently what effects does quinidine have on the digoxin?

The plasma levels of the digoxin are raised as a result of the quinidine displacing the digoxin from tissue binding sites.

❑❑ What are the major cardiac adverse effects of procainamide?

They are similar to quinidine and include "torsades de pointes."

❑❑ What are the non-cardiac adverse effects of procainamide?

Hypotension with rapid I.V. administration and a lupus erythematosus-like syndrome.

❑❑ What is the mechanism of action of disopyramide?

It is similar to quinidine but produces a greater negative inotropic effect and is a stronger anticholinergic agent.

❑❑ What are the adverse cardiac effects of disopyramide?

They are similar to quinidine, antimuscarinic adverse effects are greater than with quinidine and they also have negative inotropic activity.

❑❑ What compound will enhance the proarrhythmic activity of the Ia antiarrhythmic drugs?

Potassium.

❑❑ What class antiarrhythmic drug is lidocaine?

I_B

❑❑ How does lidocaine show selectivity?

It has pronounced effects on depolarized tissue.

❑❑ What are the therapeutic uses of lidocaine?

It is a first choice drug for ventricular arrhythmias following myocardial infarction, heart surgery and cardioconversion.

❑❑ What are the adverse reactions of lidocaine?

It has relatively few with its primary adverse effects occurring in the CNS. It can cause paresthesias and drowsiness. At toxic levels it can cause convulsions, hearing disturbances and respiratory arrest.

❏❏ **Name three other class I_B drugs besides lidocaine?**

Tocainide, mexiletine and phenytoin.

❏❏ **Give an example of a class Ic drug?**

Propafenone flecainide.

❏❏ **What is the mechanism of action of the class I_C drugs?**

They are potent sodium channel blockers. They also block K^+ channels in ventricular myocytes which prolongs the action potential.

❏❏ **What is the therapeutic use of propafenone?**

Supraventricular arrhythmias.

❏❏ **What are the adverse reactions of propafenone?**

It has proarrhythmic effects but also has a metallic taste associated with its use and causes constipation.

❏❏ **What are the drugs in Class II?**

The beta adrenergic receptor antagonists (e.g. propranolol) fall into this class.

❏❏ **How do the class II drugs work?**

They block beta adrenergic receptor regulation of K^+ and Ca^{++} channels. They also have some direct membrane effects.

❏❏ **How does propranolol differ from most of the other beta-blockers?**

It also has a direct effect on Na^+ and K^+ channels.

❏❏ **What are the therapeutic uses of the beta-blockers in the treatment of arrhythmias?**

They are used to treat ventricular arrhythmias due to exercise or emotion, they are used after an myocardial infarction to prevent recurrent infarction and for the treatment of supraventricular arrhythmias.

❏❏ **What are the adverse effects of the beta-blockers when used for the treatment of arrhythmias?**

They can worsen congestive heart failure. They can produce SA and AV block. Sudden withdrawal may also worsen angina and arrhythmias. These drugs may also cause hypotension and bronchospasm.

❏❏ **Name the class III antiarrhythmic agents?**

Bretyllium, amiodarone and sotalol

❑❑ **What ion channels do the class III drugs affect?**

They are K^+ channel blockers, therefore they block reentry arrhythmias.

❑❑ **What are the actions of bretylium on the heart?**

It produces an increased ventricular but not atrial action potential duration. It also produces an increased effective refractory period.

❑❑ **What are the therapeutic uses for bretylium?**

It is used for drug resistant ventricular fibrillations and sustained ventricular tachycardia.

❑❑ **What are the adverse effects of bretylium?**

Postural hypotension due to transient NE release. Nausea and vomiting may also occur after the IV administration of a bolus of bretylium.

❑❑ **How does amiodarone effect the heart?**

It is a K^+ channel blocker, a Na^+ and Ca^{++} channel blocker and a beta adrenergic receptor blocker.

❑❑ **What is the significant pharmacokinetic property of amiodarone?**

It has a very long half-life (1-2 months.).

❑❑ **How is amiodarone used therapeutically?**

To prevent recurrent ventricular fibrillation /ventricular tachycardia and in the treatment of supraventricular arrhythmias.

❑❑ **What are the adverse effects of amiodarone?**

Potentially fatal pulmonary toxicity, hepatic toxicity, cutaneous photosensitivity, neurologic effects and thyroid dysfunction.

❑❑ **What type of drug interactions is amiodarone involved in ?**

It increases the plasma levels of many antiarrhythmic drugs. Also if used in combination with beta-blockers or calcium antagonists it can cause sinus arrest or AV block and worsen congestive heart failure.

❑❑ **What is sotalol?**

A potassium channel blocker with effective beta-blocker activity.

❑❑ **What are the therapeutic uses of sotalol?**

It is used both for supraventricular and ventricular arrhythmias.

❏❏ What are the adverse effects of sotalol?

It can cause "torsades de pointes."

❏❏ What is esmolol and how is it used?

It is a class II blocker that is very short acting and is almost always used in the treatment of acute surgical arrhythmias.

❏❏ Which drugs are considered as Class IV antiarrhythmics?

The calcium channel blockers verapamil, diltiazem and nifedipine.

❏❏ What are the cardiac effects of the calcium channel antagonists?

They primarily effect Ca^{++} mediated slow processes like the beta-adrenergic blockers. They work best on slow tissue and they depress conduction in the AV node.

❏❏ Which of the calcium channel blockers is used therapeutically for the treatment of arrhythmias?

Verapamil.

❏❏ How are the calcium channel blockers used therapeutically?

They are first choice drugs for supraventricular tachycardia due to AV nodal reentry. They also reduce the ventricular rate in atrial flutter/fibrillation

❏❏ What are the adverse effects of verapamil?

Constipation, nausea, and peripheral edema.

❏❏ What are the contraindications for the use of verapamil?

Severe heart failure, hypotension, sick sinus syndrome, AV block, ventricular tachycardia, and Wolff-Parkinson-White syndrome combined with atrial flutter.

❏❏ Why should verapamil not be used with beta-blockers or digitalis?

There would be a danger of bradycardia or AV block.

❏❏ How does adenosine work as an antiarrhythmic drug?

It binds to adenosine receptors, which causes opening of K^+ channels and hyperpolarizes AV nodal tissue. It has opposite effects to NE, so it is acting like a beta-blocker.

❏❏ How is adenosine used therapeutically?

It is used to treat paroxysmal supraventricular tachycardia involving the AV node.

❑❑ **What is the main advantage of adenosine?**

It has a very short half-life so it is a relatively safe drug.

❑❑ **What is the mechanism of the antiarrhythmic effect of magnesium?**

The mechanism is unknown but magnesium is recognized to influence Na^+/K^+ ATPase, sodium channels, certain potassium channels and calcium channels.

❑❑ **How is magnesium used clinically for the treatment of arrhythmias?**

In patients with digitalis induced arrhythmias if hypomagnesemia is present and in some patients with torsade de pointes and in some with myocardial infarction.

❑❑ **Patients with genetically low levels of N-acetyltransferase are more prone to develop a lupus like syndrome with which drug?**

Procainamide.

DRUGS USED TO TREAT CONGESTIVE HEART FAILURE

❑❑ **What is congestive heart failure (CHF)?**

A condition where cardiac output is inadequate for the metabolic demands of the body.

❑❑ **What are the common causes of CHF?**

Myocardial infarction, hypertension, arrhythmias, and valvular disease.

❑❑ **What types of drugs can be used to treat congestive heart failure?**

Digitalis glycosides, bipyridine derivatives (amrinone and milrinone), beta-adrenergic agonists (dobutamine), vasodilators, diuretics, ACE inhibitors and beta-blockers.

❑❑ **What is the basic pathophysiology of congestive heart failure?**

There is insufficient cardiac output associated with increased blood volume and edema.

❑❑ **Which of the digitalis glycosides is most important clinically?**

Digoxin.

❑❑ **What are main differences between digoxin and digitoxin?**

Digitoxin is eliminated mainly by hepatic metabolism and it has a much longer half-life than digoxin.

❑❑ **What are the primary therapeutic uses of digitalis?**

For the treatment of congestive heart failure where its use is somewhat controversial and to treat certain arrhythmias.

❑❑ What are the direct effects of digitalis on cardiac muscle?

There is a positive inotropic effect. Digitalis increases the heart's contractile force increasing the cardiac output. This reverses the vicious cycle of congestive heart failure.

❑❑ The EKG of a patient who is receiving digoxin in the therapeutic dose range would likely show what alteration?

An increase in the PR interval, depression of the ST segment and occasional inversion of the T wave. Shortening of the QT interval is also characteristic.

❑❑ What is the mechanism of the direct effects of digitalis?

Digitalis inhibits Na^+/K^+ ATPase. This increases Na^{+i}, leading to a decreased Na^+/Ca^{++} exchanger activity, which in turn results in increased Ca^{++i}. The increased intracellular calcium results in increased contractility of the heart.

❑❑ What are the indirect effects of digitalis?

Digitalis has effects on the autonomic nervous system. It increases parasympathetic activity through an effect on the vagus.

❑❑ How are these indirect effects utilized clinically?

They are important for digitalis use in atrial arrhythmias.

❑❑ How is digitalis used in the treatment of arrhythmias?

It can reduce the ventricular rate in the presence of atrial tachycardia, atrial flutter, and atrial fibrillation.

❑❑ Explain the mechanism of the digitalis effects in arrhythmias?

At low therapeutic doses digitalis increases parasympathetic nervous system activity. It increases the effective refractory period of the AV node thus decreasing the ventricular rate in atrial flutter.

❑❑ How is digoxin eliminated?

Mainly through the kidneys.

❑❑ How is digoxin administered?

It may be given orally or IV.

❑❑ What is the major cause of digoxin toxicity?

Toxicity is most commonly due to potassium depletion, mostly when diuretics are combined with digitalis therapy.

❑❑ What types of cardiac toxicity are likely to occur from digoxin?

A variety of arrhythmias occur as a result of increased automaticity, triggered activity and reentry. They result from both direct and indirect effects on multiple regions of the heart.

❑❑ What other toxicities are associated with digoxin use?

GI related (anorexia, nausea/vomiting and sometimes diarrhea) and neurological/visual effects (headache, confusion, aphasia and delirium; altered color perception).

❑❑ What is the treatment for digitalis toxicity?

Monitor the EKG, determine and correct potassium and digitalis levels. Lidocaine can be used for digitalis induced ventricular arrhythmias and in extreme cases digibind antibodies can be used.

❑❑ What types of drug interactions occur with digitalis?

Potassium depleting diuretics lower potassium levels and increase digoxin toxicity; quinidine, verapamil and amiodarone increase digoxin concentrations.

❑❑ How do the bipyridine compounds increase myocardial contractility?

They don't inhibit Na^+/K^+ ATPase or activate adrenoreceptors. They appear to increase inward clacium flux in the heart during the action potential and alter the intracellular movements of calcium by influencing the sarcoplasmic reticulum.

❑❑ What type of toxicity is associated with the use of the bipyridine compounds?

A relatively high incidence of nausea and vomiting; thrombocytopenia and liver enzyme changes.

❑❑ Wich adrenergic receptor agonists are frequently used in patients with heart failure?

Dobutamine and dopamine.

TREATMENT OF ANGINA

❑❑ How do you define angina pectoris?

The severe chest pain that occurs when there is inadequate coronary blood flow to supply the oxygen required by the heart.

❑❑ What is the basic problem in angina pectoris?

An imbalance between the oxygen requirement of the heart and the oxygen supplied to it by the coronary vessels. In classical angina the imbalance occurs when the myocardial oxygen requirement increases as during exercise and the coronary blood flow doesn't increase proportionately.

❏❏ What are the three types of angina pectoris?

Chronic stable angina (classic), variant (Prinzmetal's) angina and unstable angina.

❏❏ What are the differences between these three types of angina?

In chronic stable angina there is the presence of atheromatous obstruction in coronary arteries. In variant angina there is a coronary artery spasm, and in unstable angina there is the presence of thrombin near atherosclerotic plaques.

❏❏ Which type of angina is most common?

Classic angina is the most common accounting for about 90% of the cases.

❏❏ What are the therapeutic goals for each type of angina?

In stable angina we want to increase myocardium perfusion or decrease oxygen demand. In variant angina we want to prevent vasospasm and in unstable angina we want to correct the tendency to form thrombi.

❏❏ What are the organic nitrates?

Nitric and nitrous acid esters of polyalcohols.

❏❏ What compound are the organic nitrates converted to in vascular tissue?

Nitric oxide.

❏❏ What is the mechanism of action of the nitrates to relieve angina?

They relax vascular smooth muscle through conversion into nitric oxide (NO) and subsequent elevation of intracellular cGMP. The increased cGMP results in myosin light chain dephosphorylation (relaxation).

❏❏ What are the vascular effects of nitroglycerin?

Relaxation of all veins and arteries (especially venous). There is a decreased ventricular preload, a dilation of coronary arteries, decreased mechanical work and oxygen consumption and increased exercise tolerance.

❏❏ What are the cardiac effects of nitroglycerin?

There are no direct inotropic or chronotropic effects but a reflex tachycardia may occur.

❏❏ Are other smooth muscles effected by nitroglycerin?

There is relaxation of bronchi and the GI and biliary tracts.

❑❑ Is platelet aggregation effected by nitroglycerin?

Yes, there is an increase in cGMP and a decreased aggregation.

❑❑ How is nitroglycerin metabolized?

By hepatic organic nitrate reductase. There is extensive first pass metabolism of nitroglycerin in the liver. Therefore it is commonly given sublingually or through the use of a transdermal patch.

❑❑ How is nitroglycerin administered?

Sublingually, orally, transdermal, buccal and IV.

❑❑ What is the advantage of sublingual administration of nitroglycerin?

A very rapid action, and lack of first pass metabolism.

❑❑ When is the IV route used for nitroglycerin?

In intensive care facilities.

❑❑ What adverse effects are associated with the use of nitroglycerin?

The most common sign is a throbbing headache. Other effects include orthostatic hypotension, reflex tachycardia and flushing.

❑❑ What is meant by tolerance to nitroglycerin?

When you get a decreased or lack of effect.

❑❑ When does tolerance occur to nitroglycerin?

After long term administration of the drug.

❑❑ What is the mechanism of the tolerance to nitroglycerin?

It is due to decreased guanylate cyclase activation, ANS compensatory mechanisms and salt and water retention.

❑❑ How is the tolerance to nitroglycerin reversed?

By stopping the drug for 8 hours.

❑❑ What are the therapeutic uses of nitroglycerin?

Acute anginal attacks, and maintenance therapy to prevent attacks.

❑❑ How does isosorbide dinitrate and other nitrates differ from nitroglycerin?

They have similar effects to nitroglycerin but are slower acting and are more commonly used for maintenance therapy.

❑❑ How is amyl nitrate administered?

It is inhaled.

❑❑ What are the four calcium channel blockers used to treat angina?

Dihydropyridines (nifedipine, nimodipine.), diltiazem, verapamil and bepridil.

❑❑ What is the mechanism of action of the calcium channel blockers in angina?

They produce blockade of L-type calcium channels and a marked decrease in transmembrane calcium current.

❑❑ What are the cardiovascular effects of nifedipine?

A reduction in peripheral vascular resistance, a decreased afterload, dilatation of coronary arteries and weak cardiac effects.

❑❑ What are the major toxic effects associated with the use of nifedipine?

Vasodilatation (headache, hypotension, dizziness); skin rash, sleepiness, G,I. effects and aggravation of angina at high doses.

❑❑ What are the therapeutic uses of nifedipine?

Angina and hypertension.

❑❑ What is the advantage of diltiazem over the other calcium channel blockers?

It has a low incidence of side effects.

❑❑ What are the vascular effects of verapamil?

A reduction in peripheral vascular resistance; decreased afterload and dilatation of coronary arteries.

❑❑ What effects does verapamil have on the heart?

Negative inotropism, chronotropism, and dromotropism. There is a reduction in oxygen requirement and autonomic reflex effects are blunted.

❑❑ What are the therapeutic uses of verapamil?

Angina, hypertension and arrhythmias.

❒❒ What are the adverse effects of verapamil?

Cardiac depression and commonly constipation.

❒❒ Why is the use of verapamil with beta blockers contraindicated ?

Both produce negative chronotropic and inotropic effects.

❒❒ What is the major difference in the action of verapamil compared to nifedipine?

With nifedipine you see an ANS reflex effect due to a lack of calcium channel blockage in the heart while you don't with verapamil.

❒❒ What is the mechanism of action of the beta-adrenergic blockers in angina?

They antagonize the effects of beta-adrenergic receptor agonists, cause negative inotropism, negative chronotropism and reduce myocardial oxygen demands.

❒❒ Which are the lipophilic beta-blockers?

Propranolol, metoprolol, and timolol.

❒❒ What advantage do the lipophilic beta-blockers have?

They cross the blood brain barrier and are readily absorbed after oral administration.

❒❒ Which are the hydrophilic beta-blockers ?

Atenolol and nadolol.

❒❒ What properties do the lipophilic beta-blockers have?

They do not cross the blood brain barrier and are excreted by the kidney.

❒❒ What is the distinguishing feature about nadolol?

It has a long duration of action (up to 24 hours).

❒❒ What is the advantage of the cardioselective beta-blockers?

They have reduced aggravating effects in pulmonary disease and peripheral vascular disease.

❒❒ How are the beta-blockers used therapeutically?

They are used in angina in combination with nitrates and they are also used in hypertension and certain other diseases.

❒❒ What drugs are used to treat variant angina?

Organic nitrates and calcium channel blocking agents.

❑❑ **What drugs are used to treat unstable angina?**

Nitroglycerin (I.V.), verapamil or nifedipine with beta-adrenergic receptor antagonists, or beta adrenergic receptor antagonists.

❑❑ **Why is the use of sildenafil contraindicated with organic nitrates?**

You may get an extreme lowering of blood pressure.

TREATMENT OF HYPERTENSION

❑❑ **How are the thiazide diuretics used in the treatment of hypertension?**

They provide adequate therapy for mild to moderate hypertension. They can be used alone or in combination with sympatholytics or vasodilators in more severe hypertension.

❑❑ **What are the hemodynamic effects of the thiazides?**

They reduce blood volume, reduce cardiac output, and peripheral resistance may increase.

❑❑ **Where does clonidine act?**

Centrally at $alpha_2$ adrenergic receptors.

❑❑ **What are the hemodynamic effects of clonidine?**

There is decreased heart rate, decreased vascular resistance but renal blood flow is maintained.

❑❑ **What are the adverse effects of clonidine?**

Dry mouth, sedation and impotence.

❑❑ **What is the clonidine withdrawal syndrome?**

A syndrome of headache, tremors, abdominal pain and tachycardia followinh abrupt withdrawal.

❑❑ **What is the mechanism of action of methyldopa?**

It is a false transmitter with similar effects to clonidine.

❑❑ **What are the adverse effects of methydopa?**

Sedation, CNS effects and a positive Coombs test.

❒❒ **How does terazosin work?**

It blocks $alpha_1$ adrenergic receptors.

❒❒ **What are the hemodynamic effects of terazosin?**

Arterial pressure is reduced, fluid and salt are retained.

❒❒ **What are the pharmacokinetic differences between terazosin and other selective α_1-adrenergic receptor blockers?**

Terazosin has a higher oral bioavailability and a long half-life of about 12 hours.

❒❒ **What are the toxic effects of terazosin?**

There is a first dose effect like prazosin and the other adverse effects also are similar to prazosin.

❒❒ **How does propanolol lower blood pressure?**

It is a beta adrenergic receptor antagonist.

❒❒ **What are the cardiovascular effects of propranolol?**

It decreases heart rate and cardiac output. There is a slowly developing reduction in blood pressure.

❒❒ **What other beta-adrenergic receptor blockers beside propranolol are often used to lower blood pressure?**

Atenolol, pindolol, and labetalol.

❒❒ **Which one of these beta-adrenergic receptor blockers also blocks alpha-receptors?**

Labetalol.

❒❒ **What advantage is it to being a selective blocker?**

There is a reduced likelihood of bronchospasm or coldness of the extremities.

❒❒ **What is the mechanism of action of hydralazine?**

It produces arteriolar dilatation by an unknown mechanism.

❒❒ **What are the adverse effects of hydralazine?**

Headache, sweating, and reflex tachycardia.

❒❒ **How does sodium nitroprusside lower blood pressure?**

It dilates arterial and venous vessels. Its action occurs as a result of activation of guanylate cyclase either as a result of release of nitric oxide or by direct stimulation of the enzyme.

❒❒ How is nitroprusside used clinically?

In hypertensive emergencies as it rapidly lowers blood pressure.

❒❒ What are the toxic effects of nitroprusside?

The most serious toxicity is cyanide accumulation; metabolic acidosis, arrhythmias, excessive hypotension and death have resulted.

❒❒ How does diazoxide work?

It dilates arteries. It opens potassium channels and stabilizes the membrane potential at the resting level causing vasodilation.

❒❒ What are the therapeutic uses of diazoxide?

It is used to treat hypertensive emergencies.

❒❒ What types of toxicity does diazoxide have?

Excessive hypotension is the most significant toxicity from diazoxide. Such hypotension has resulted in stroke and myocardial infarction.

❒❒ How does nifedipine lower blood pressure?

It blocks calcium channels in the vasculature but not in the heart.

❒❒ What is the advantage of nifedipine in the treatment of high blood pressure?

It is more selective as a vasodilator and has less cardiac depressant effects than verapamil and diltiazem.

❒❒ What is the mechanism by which the angiotensin converting enzyme (ACE) inhibitors lower blood pressure?

They inhibit the enzyme forming angiotensin II, a potent vasoconstrictor. They also may block metabolism of bradykinin prolonging its action.

❒❒ Name three ACE inhibitors.

Captopril, Enalapril and Lisinopril.

❒❒ What are the hemodynamic effects of captopril and other ACE inhibitors?

Vascular resistance is lowered, with little effect on heart rate and cardiac output.

❑❑ What are the adverse effects of the ACE inhibitors?

Acute renal failure, dry cough and hyperkalemia when used with potassium-sparing diuretics.

❑❑ How does enalapril differ from captopril?

Enalapril is a prodrug, which is converted to an ACE inhibitor.

❑❑ Name two angiotensin receptor antagonists?

Losartan and valsartan.

❑❑ What is the mechanism of action of losartan?

It is a potent and specific competitive antagonist of angiotensin AT_1 receptors. It inhibits angiotensin II mediated contraction of vascular smooth muscle. It reduces blood pressure in the renovascular system and genetic hypertension. It has no effect on bradykinin metabolism.

❑❑ What are the adverse effects of losartan and other angiotensin receptor antagonists?

Hypotension and GI effects. No cough or angioedema is produced, however.

DRUGS FOR TREATMENT OF HYPERLIPIDEMIA

❑❑ What is a lipoprotein?

Spherical or ellipsoid particles composed of a core of non-polar lipid and this is surrounded by protein and polar lipid.

❑❑ Name the 6 groups of lipoproteins?

LDL, VLDL, chylomicrons, chylomicron remnants, HDL and IDL's.

❑❑ What are the basic causes of hyperlipoproteinemias?

There are primary hyperlipoproteinemias, which are due to basic genetic defects and secondary hyperlipoproteinemias, which are due to some other metabolic disorder.

❑❑ Which lipoproteins are considered atherogenic?

LDL, VLDL and IDL.

❑❑ Which lipoproteins are considered antiatherogenic?

HDL.

❑❑ What dietary strategies can be tried to lower lipoprotein levels?

Decrease cholesterol and saturated fat intake, increase the amount of soluble fiber and fish oil supplements.

❑❑ How do the statins effect plasma lipids and lipoproteins?

They lower LDLs mainly but also lower TG concentrations. HDL concentrations increase.

❑❑ Which statin is currently the most effective in lowering LDL levels?

Atorvastatin.

❑❑ Name five statins used to lower lipid levels?

Lovastatin, pravastatin, atorvastatin, cervistatin, simvastatin and fluvastatin.

❑❑ What is the main difference among the different statins?

They have differences mainly in pharmacokinetic parameters.

❑❑ What is the mechanism of action of the statins?

They are competitive inhibitors of HMG CoA reductase, the rate limiting enzyme in cholesterol synthesis. This leads to a compensatory increase in hepatic LDL receptors and an increased removal of LDL particles from the circulation.

❑❑ When are the statins best given?

In the evening as the maximum cholesterol synthesis occurs early in the morning.

❑❑ How does the body handle the statins?

They are mostly metabolised by the liver cytochrome P450 enzymes.

❑❑ What are the clinical uses of the statins?

They are considered first line therapy for hypercholesterolemia due to elevated LDL especially Type IIa hypercholesterolemia.

❑❑ What are the common adverse reactions associated with statin use?

GI irritation, headache and rash are common. Elevation of liver enzymes may occur. Muscle pain also occurs.

❑❑ What precaution is advisable when using lovastatin?

Periodic liver serum transaminase levels should be taken.

❑❑ **What type of drug interactions may occur with the statins?**

Several of them are metabolized by the cytochrome P450 3A4 isoenzyme so combining them with other drugs that inhibit this enzyme may increase their toxicity.

❑❑ **Why are the statins contraindicated in pregnancy?**

The long-term effects are not known and they have been shown to be teratogenic in animal studies.

❑❑ **What drugs belong to the fibric acid group of antilipidemics?**

Gemfibrozil, fenofibrate and clofibrate are available in the U.S.

❑❑ **What groups of lipoproteins do the fibric acids mainly affect?**

VLDL concentrations are lowered about 40-55%.

❑❑ **What happens to HDL levels after giving these drugs?**

HDL cholesterol is increased.

❑❑ **What is their mechanism of action?**

The primary effect is to increase the activity of lipoprotein lipase, which will promote the catabolism of VLDL levels. They may also reduce the incorporation of long-chain fatty acids into newly formed triglycerides thus reducing VLDL synthesis and release from the liver.

❑❑ **How are the fibric acid derivatives used clinically?**

They are used in patients with elevated triglyceride levels, such as patients with types III, IV and V hyperlipidemias.

❑❑ **What are the adverse reactions of the fibric acid drugs?**

GI disturbances are frequent and skin rash occurs with some. Clofibrate has caused arrhythmias.

❑❑ **What is the danger of using fibric acid derivatives with the statins?**

There is an increased risk of rhabdomyolysis.

❑❑ **What are the two principal bile acids binding resins available?**

Colestipol and cholestyramine.

❑❑ **What is the mechanism of action of the bile acid binding resins?**

They bind bile acids in the intestine and prevent their reabsorption. This lowers the normal feedback inhibition of the enzyme converting cholesterol to bile acids and results in increased breakdown of hepatic cholesterol. The increased cholesterol breakdown leads to an increase in HMG CoA reductase and an increased number of LDL receptors.

❑❑ What lipids are effected by the bile acid binding resins?

LDL levels are decreased to a small degree and there is a modest increase in HDL levels.

❑❑ Are the bile acid binding resins well absorbed?

They are not absorbed after oral administration.

❑❑ How are the bile acid binding resins used clinically?

In type II hypercholesterolemia, where there is a LDL receptor defect.

❑❑ What groups of drugs are they best used combination with?

The statins.

❑❑ What adverse effects do these bile acid binding resins produce?

GI effects are most common, and include constipation, belching and flatulence. Also mild steatorrhea can develop because they can bind many anions, resulting in increased fecal excretion of long-chain fatty acids.

❑❑ What kinds of drug-drug interactions occur with these drugs?

They interact with many different drugs if given concurrently. This results from a binding to the drugs as they bind bile acids. Among the drugs interacting include digitalis, thiazides, warfarin, vancomycin, thyroxine and aspirin.

❑❑ How can these drug interactions be avoided?

Other drugs should be given 1-2 hours before or 4 hours after the bile acid binding resins.

❑❑ What is the mechanism of action of probucol?

It is an antioxidant.

❑❑ What are the adverse effects of probucol?

GI disturbances and cardiotoxicity.

❑❑ What effect does nicotinic acid (niacin) have on blood lipid levels?

It rapidly lowers VLDL and more slowly lowers LDL cholesterol. There are also mild to moderate increases in HDL cholesterol.

❑❑ Through what mechanism does nicotinic acid work?

It decreases the synthesis of VLDL, which in turn results in decreased production of its daughter particles IDL and LDL and increased HDL levels. It also lowers VLDL through several diverse mechanisms including inhibition of lipolysis in adipose tissue, decreased esterification of triglycerides in liver and increased activity of lipoprotein lipase.

❑❑ **How is nicotinic acid used clinically?**

It is used in all types of lipoprotein disorders. It is usually used in combination with other antilipidemic drugs.

❑❑ **What adverse effects are seen very soon after administering nicotinic acid?**

Flushing and itching.

❑❑ **What is the cause of the vasodilation produced by nicotinic acid?**

Nicotinic acid stimulates production of prostaglandins.

❑❑ **How can the flushing and itching be prevented or ameliorated?**

By using aspirin or antihistamines.

❑❑ **What other adverse effect is common with nicotinic acid?**

GI disturbances.

❑❑ **How can the GI toxicity of nicotinic acid be decreased?**

Take the niacin with meals or start with low doses.

❑❑ **What are some of the more severe toxicities associated with nicotinic acid use?**

Hepatotoxicity, activation of peptic ulcer, hyperglycemia and decreased glucose tolerance and hyperuricemia.

❑❑ **What combination of drugs would you use to treat severe hypertriglyceridemia?**

Gemfibrozil and nicotinic acid.

TREATMENT OF ANEMIAS

❑❑ **A deficiency of vitamin B12 or folic acid results in defective synthesis of what?**

DNA.

❑❑ **What are the early signs of B12 deficiency?**

Megaloblastic or pernicious anemia.

❑❑ **What are the sources of B12 in man?**

Soil microorganisms, that contaminate vegetables and meat.

❑❑ **What are the active forms of vitamin B12?**

Deoxyadenosylcobalamin and methylcobalamin.

❑❑ **What are the forms available for therapeutic use?**

Cyanocobalamin and hydroxycobalamin.

❑❑ **What is intrinsic factor?**

A 59 kDA protein secreted by the parietal cells of the stomach.

❑❑ **What is the function of intrinsic factor?**

It is necessary for B12 absorption.

❑❑ **What causes B12 deficiency in humans?**

Malabsorption of B12 due either to lack of intrinsic factor or to loss or malfunction of the specific absorptive mechanisms in the distal ileum.

❑❑ **Where is excess B12 stored?**

In the liver.

❑❑ **What is the function of folic acid?**

It is necessary for the formation of folate cofactors. These are essential for one-carbon transfer reactions, which in turn are necessary for DNA synthesis.

❑❑ **What is the clinical use of folic acid?**

To treat or prevent deficiencies of folic acid.

❑❑ **What are the consequences of B12 and folic acid deficiency on the nervous system?**

Neurological damage.

❑❑ **What are the hematopoietic consequences of B12 and folic acid deficiency?**

Megaloblastic anemia.

❑❑ **Will folic acid correct the anemia due to vitamin B12 deficiency?**

Yes.

❑❑ **Will folic acid correct the neurological damage due to B12 deficiency?**

No.

❑❑ **What causes folate deficiency?**

It results from diseases of the small intestine, alcoholism and treatment with inhibitors of dihydrofolate reductase.

❑❑ **How is folic acid administered?**

It is given orally. It is well absorbed and non-toxic even at high doses.

❑❑ **Is folic acid ever given parenterally?**

For the acutely ill, it may be given IM.

❑❑ **How is vitamin B12 administered?**

IM injection is safe and must be continued for life.

❑❑ **Why is B12 not given IV?**

It may cause severe allergic reactions such as anaphylaxis.

❑❑ **What is the most common cause of nutritional anemia?**

Iron deficiency.

❑❑ **Where is the major location of essential iron?**

In hemoglobin.

❑❑ **The reduction of hemoglobin synthesis results in what type of anemia?**

Hypochromic microcytic anemia.

❑❑ **How is iron absorbed?**

Iron is transported across the intestinal mucosa by active transport. It is absorbed as ferrous iron and is converted to ferric iron within the mucosal cell.

❑❑ **How is iron transported?**

Via transferrin.

❑❑ **Where is iron stored?**

In the reticuloendothelial system, hepatocytes and muscle.

❑❑ How is iron excreted?

There is no mechanism for iron excretion.

❑❑ What are the causes of iron deficiency?

Inadequate dietary intake, excessive blood loss and inhibition of absorption.

❑❑ What are the clinical indications for the use of iron?

Iron deficiency anemia.

❑❑ How is iron administered?

Orally or parenterally (IV or IM).

❑❑ What preparations are used orally?

A variety of salts, including ferrous sulfate, fumarate and gluconate. Only ferrous salts should be used.

❑❑ What are the side effects of oral iron therapy

Heartburn, nausea, constipation and diarrhea.

❑❑ When is iron given parenterally?

In patients with documented iron deficiency unable to tolerate or absorb oral iron and patients with extensive chronic blood loss who can't be maintained with oral iron alone.

❑❑ What form is parenteral iron in?

Iron dextran. A stable complex of ferric hydroxide and low-M.W. dextran.

❑❑ How is iron given parenterally?

It is given by deep I.M. injection or by I.V. infusion.

❑❑ What are the side effects of IM iron?

When given intramuscularly there is local tissue staining and pain, which can be avoided with IV injection. However, both parenteral sites may cause hypersensitivity reactions.

❑❑ How is iron poisoning treated?

With iron chelation therapy using deferoxamine.

ANTICOAGULANTS, THROMBOLITICS AND ANTIPLATELET DRUGS

❑❑ **What is a thrombus?**

It is a clot that forms in a blood vessel and which can completely block that vessel.

❑❑ **What two drugs are commonly used as anticoagulants?**

Heparin and coumadin.

❑❑ **What is heparin?**

Heparin is a heterogeneous mixture of sulfated mucopolysaccharides.

❑❑ **How does heparin normally exist in the body?**

It is normally found complexed to histamine in mast cells.

❑❑ **What is low M.W. heparin?**

Low M.W. heparins (1-10 kDa; mean 4.5 kDa) are isolated from standard heparin. Low M.W. heparins (enoxaparin and dalteparin) differ from standard heparin in both pharmacokinetics and mechanism of action.

❑❑ **How is heparin administered?**

By continuous or intermittent IV infusion or SC injection.

❑❑ **What is the onset of action of heparin?**

Very rapid, 1-2 minutes.

❑❑ **What is the mechanism of action of heparin?**

It must bind to heparin cofactor or antithrombin III. This binding greatly increases the rate of thrombin-antithrombin III interaction and inhibits the proteolytic activity of thrombin. Also inhibited are factors Xa, and to a lesser extent factors Ixa, XIa, XIIa and kallikrein.

❑❑ **How does low M.W. heparin work?**

There is little activity on thrombin inhibition. The major mechanism is inhibition of factor Xa by antithrombin III.

❑❑ **What is hirudin?**

A direct inhibitor of thrombin that addresses some limitations of heparin therapy. It is a protein isolated from the leech.

❑❑ **When heparin is used what measurement is used to adjust the dose?**

Activated partial thromboplastin time (aPTT). One wants to maintain an activated PTT of 1.5-2.5 times the control value.

❑❑ **What measurement is used to adjust the dose of coumarin?**

One wants to obtain an International Normalized Ratio of 2-3.

❑❑ **What is the major toxic effect of heparin?**

Bleeding.

❑❑ **What will reverse the effects of heparin?**

Slow I.V. infusion of protamine sulfate.

❑❑ **How does protamine work?**

Protamine binds heparin tightly and prevents the interaction of heparin with antithrombin III.

❑❑ **What other side effects may be associated with heparin use?**

Thrombocytopenia, abnormal hepatic function tests, inhibition of aldosterone synthesis, nausea, vomiting, headache, lacrimation and fever.

❑❑ **How can the thrombocytopenia produced by heparin be reversed?**

Discontinue the heparin.

❑❑ **What is warfarin and where does it come from?**

Warfarin is a synthetic derivative of dicumarol. It can cause disease in cattle that have ingested spoiled sweet clover.

❑❑ **How is warfarin given?**

It is given orally.

❑❑ **Does warfarin have a rapid action like heparin?**

No, its anticoagulant action is delayed and appears 36-72 hours after the start of therapy.

❑❑ **What is the mechanism of warfarin's anticoagulant action?**

Warfarin inhibits the reduction of vitamin K and decreases the concentration of the active form of vitamin K.

❑❑ What will reverse the action of warfarin?

Vitamin K.

❑❑ How does vitamin K work?

Vitamin K provides functional coagulation factors and bypasses the metabolic block that results in the synthesis of defective coagulation factors.

❑❑ How long does it take vitamin K to reverse the effects of warfarin?

Up to 24 hours or longer.

❑❑ What can you do for immediate restoration of hemostasis in the case of warfarin overdose?

Transfusion of fresh frozen plasma.

❑❑ What is the major toxicity of warfarin?

Bleeding.

❑❑ What is the cause of the numerable drug-drug interactions with warfarin?

It is 99% bound to plasma albumin, and it is inactivated by transformation to inactive metabolites. Therefore displacement from albumin and/or drugs that alter cytochrome P450 metabolism can interact with warfarin.

❑❑ Is heparin contraindicated in pregnancy?

It does not cross the placenta and may be used if necessary.

❑❑ Is warfarin contraindicated in pregnancy?

Yes, it causes birth defects and abortion if given during pregnancy.

❑❑ Is thrombolytic therapy specific?

Thrombolytic therapy degrades fibrin but the general activation of this system causes nonspecific lysis of both pathological clots and beneficial clots at the site of injury.

❑❑ What do thrombolytic agents do?

They are plasminogen activators. They convert the zymogen plasminogen to the active enzyme plasmin. Plasmin acts to degrade the fibrin framework of the clot.

❑❑ What is streptokinase?

A 47kDa protein isolated from hemolytic streptococci.

❑❑ How does streptokinase work?

It forms an equimolar complex with plasminogen. The resulting change in plasminogen activates the serine protease activity and converts other plasminogen molecules to plasmin.

❑❑ What is anistreplase?

A 1:1 complex of streptokinase and lys-plasminogen, which is anisoylated at the active serine. The slow hydrolysis of the acyl group occurs and converts the inactive lys-plasminogen to active lys-plasminogen which can then activate plasminogen to plasmin.

❑❑ How does tPA work?

It is a 68kDa protein that has serine protease activity. It is a physiologic plasmingen activator. It binds to fibrin and activates fibrin bound plasminogen better than free plasminogen.

❑❑ What is urokinase and how does it work?

It is a 54 kDa.protein that is a serine protease and converts plasminogen to plasmin.

❑❑ How are thrombolytic agents administered?

They are given by IV or by intracoronary infusion.

❑❑ What are aminocaproic acid and tranexamic acid?

Lysine analog inhibitors of fibrinolysis.

❑❑ How do aminocaproic acid and tranexamic acid work?

They inhibit fibrinolysis by binding and blocking the lysine binding site on plasminogen tha tis used to bind fibrin.

❑❑ What is the major toxicity of all thrombolytic therapy?

Bleeding and hemorrhage.

❑❑ When is thrombolytic therapy contraindicated?

In patients that have active bleeding or hemorrhagic disorders, surgery within the last 10 days, a history of hypertension or previous intracranial cerebrovascular disease.

❑❑ What are antiplatelet drugs used for?

To prevent thrombosis.

❑❑ What antiplatelet drugs are available?

Aspirin, ticlopidine and dipyridamole.

❏❏ **How does aspirin work as an antiplatelet drug?**

It inhibits thromboxane A2 synthesis irreversibly and inhibits platelet aggregation.

❏❏ **What dose is maximally effective?**

Low doses (160-325 mg/day) are maximally effective. Higher doses do not produce better inhibition but do increase toxicity and bleeding.

❏❏ **Is routine use of aspirin recommended in healthy adults?**

No, but it may be considered in patients at high risk for coronary disease.

❏❏ **When is antiplatelet therapy called for?**

It is strongly recommended for patients having angina pectoris, acute M.I., transient ischemic attacks, and chronic vascular disease.

❏❏ **When is ticlopidine used?**

In patients who can't tolerate aspirin.

❏❏ **What is the mechanism of action of ticlopidine?**

It is not completely understood but it is thought to inhibit the action of ADP on platelets.

❏❏ **How does dipyridamole work?**

It increases platelet cAMP by inhibiting cyclic nucleotide phosphodiesterase and inhibits platelet aggregation.

❏❏ **How is dipyridamole used?**

It is ineffective when used alone. It is usually used in combination with warfarin to prevent thromboemboli formation in prosthetic heart valves.

ANTITUSSIVES

❏❏ **What is an antitussive?**

An agent that prevents cough.

❏❏ **When would you use an antitussive?**

Antitussives have a limited role. They are used in acute respiratory tract infections where cough disrupts sleep. In this case antitussives may be useful.

❏❏ **How do opiates work to suppress cough?**

They decrease the sensitivity of the CNS to peripheral stimuli and decrease mucosal secretion.

❑❑ Name some opiates used as antitussives?

Codeine, hydrocodone and hydromorphone.

❑❑ What is dextromorphan?

A synthetic derivative of codeine. It is the d isomer of the codeine analog levorphanol.

❑❑ What is the mechanism of action of dextromethorphan?

It suppresses the response of the cough center. However, unlike the L isomer it has no analgesic or addictive properties and does not act through opioid receptors.

❑❑ What is benzonatate?

It is an antitussive. It is a long chain polyglycol derivative chemically related to procaine.

❑❑ How does benzonatate work as an antitussive?

It has an action on the stretch or cough receptors in the lung as well as by a central mechanism.

ANTIMICROBIAL DRUGS

❑❑ **Define antibiotic?**

Chemicals produced by microorganisms and that inhibit the growth of or kill other microorganisms.

❑❑ **Define selective toxicity?**

The ability of a chemotherapeutic agent to affect a foreign organism without affecting the host.

❑❑ **What are the advantages of combination therapy?**

Synergism, ability to avoid resistance, ability to treat mixed infections, and ability to treat serious infections of unknown etiology.

❑❑ **What are the disadvantages of combination therapy?**

Increased toxicity, increased cost, increased likelihood of superinfections, antagonism between bactericidal and bacteriostatic agents.

❑❑ **What is meant by the term fixed dose combinations?**

Two or more antibiotics put together in one dosage form without a rationale basis for the dosage used.

❑❑ **What is meant by the postantibiotic effect?**

Persistent suppression of bacterial growth after brief expsure to an antimicrobial agent.

❑❑ **During treatment of a primary infection with an antibiotic the appearance of a secondary infection as a result of alteration in the associated bacterial flora is referred to as a ____________?**

Superinfection.

❑❑ **How is a superinfection treated?**

The original antibiotic should be stopped and treatment begun with an antibiotic effective against the developing superinfection.

❑❑ **What are two major genetic causes of antibiotic mediated resistance?**

Plasmid alterations and chromosomal mutations.

❑❑ Which is the more common clinically, plasmid or chromosomally mediated resistance?

Plasmid mediated.

❑❑ Why is plasmid mediated resistance more common clinically?

There is transmission to different species and genera. Chromosome mutations cause derangements in the bacteria and inhibit growth.

❑❑ What is meant by the term cross resistance?

When there is resistance to one drug in a particular class there is resistance to all the drugs.

❑❑ How can resistance to antibiotics best be avoided?

By the careful and judicious use of antibiotics, by using combination therapy in some infections and by using adequate doses of the antibiotic.

❑❑ What are the uses of prophylactic chemotherapy?

To protect against an infection caused by a specific organism, before certain surgical procedures and in cancer and immunosuppressed patients.

❑❑ What is the difference between a bacteriostatic and bactericidal antibiotic?

A bacteriostatic drug inhibits bacterial growth while a bactericidal agent will kill the bacteria.

❑❑ What is the mechanism of action of the sulfonamides?

Inhibition of folic acid synthesis mainly by competitive inhibition of the enzime dihydropteroate synthetase.

❑❑ What is the natural metabolite that the sulfonamides compete with?

PABA (p-aminobenzoic acid).

❑❑ Which is the most common adverse effect associated with the use of sulfonamides?

Allergic reactions especially skin rashes

❑❑ What are the advantages of combining sulfamethoxazole with trimethoprim?

Bactericidal effect; decreased resistance; less toxicity and an extended spectrum of activity

❑❑ What is the ideal ratio of sulfamethoxazole : trimethoprim that is present in this combination?

5:1, this ratio allows approximately equal amounts of both drugs to be available.

❑❑ How are the sulfonamides metabolized?

By acetylation of the amino group.

❑❑ What are the disadvantages of the acetylated form compared to the parent sulfonamide?

The acetylated form is less soluble, lacks antibacterial activity and is more toxic.

❑❑ Why are sulfonamides contraindicated in pregnancy and lactation?

Because of the possibility of kernicterus whereby bilirubin is displaced from protein binding sites and goes to the CNS in the very young.

❑❑ How can the crystalluria caused by some of the sulfonamides be prevented?

By using triple sulfonamides (independent solubility), by using the newer soluble sulfonamides and by alkalinization of the urine.

❑❑ What is the most common therapeutic use of the sulfonamides alone?

Acute, simple urinary tract infections (UTIs).

❑❑ What is the site of action of trimethoprim?

Inhibition of bacterial dihydrofolate reductase.

❑❑ What drug can prevent the bone marrow suppression associated with use of trimethoprim-sulfonamide combinations?

Leucovorin (citrovorum factor, folinic acid).

❑❑ What are the major uses of the trimethoprim-sulfamethoxazole combination?

Chronic and recurrent urinary tract infections, bronchitis, *Peumocystis carinii* pneumonia and travelers diarrhea.

❑❑ What structural feature do the penicillins, cephalosporins, carbapenems and monobactams all share in common?

The β-lactam ring.

❑❑ What is the basic mechanism of action of the penicillins?

Inhibition of cell wall synthesis.

❑❑ Which is the enzyme inhibited by penicillins that results in inhibition of cell wall synthesis?

Transpeptidase.

❒❒ How do the penicillins actually kill bacteria?

By inhibiting the release of murein hydrolases (autolysins).

❒❒ What is the most common cause of clinical resistance to the penicillins?

Increased production of the enzyme penicillinase

❒❒ For each of the following infections which penicillin is best used to treat the patient?

A streptococcal infection?

Penicillin G.

Acute otitis media?

Amoxicillin or ampicillin.

Serious pseudomonas infections?

Ticarcillin, piperacillin.

An infection due to staphylococcus aureus?

Cloxacillin, Oxacillin, Nafcillin.

Syphilis?

Benzathine penicillin G.

Prophylaxis of rheumatic fever?

Penicillin V.

Name the penicillinase resistant penicillins?

Methicillin, nafcillin, oxacillin, dicloxacillin and cloxacillin.

❒❒ Which of these penicillinase resistant penicillins can only be given parenterally?

Methicillin and nafcillin.

❒❒ How are methicillin-resistant *Staphylococcus aureus* infections treated?

With vancomycin.

❑❑ **For the treatment of serious infections caused by *Pseudomonas aeruginosa,* an antipseudomonal penicillin is usually combined with?**

An aminoglycoside such as gentamicin or tobramycin.

❑❑ **Give some examples of anti-pseudomonal penicillins?**

Mezlocillin, ticarcillin, carbenicillin, azlocillin and piperacillin.

❑❑ **Are the anti-pseudomonal penicillins inactivated by penicillinase?**

Yes.

❑❑ **How are these antipseudomonal penicillins administered?**

Parenterally, as they are unstable in gastric acid.

❑❑ **What two repository preparations of penicillin are available?**

Penicillin G procaine and penicillin G benzathine.

❑❑ **What is meant by the term repository preparation?**

A preparation of penicillin that provides low but long-lasting concentrations of penicillin. They are injected IM and slowly dissolve from the IM sites.

❑❑ **What is the major adverse effect associated with penicillin use?**

Hypersensitivity reactions.

❑❑ **What toxicity is likely to seen with the antipseudomonal penicillins, ticarcillin and carbenicllin?**

Platelet dysfunction.

❑❑ **What toxicity is limits the use of methicillin?**

Renal toxicity.

❑❑ **What toxicities are associated with ampicillin?**

The incidence of rash is high in some patients. Also pseudomembranous colitis may occur.

❑❑ **What is the purpose of combining clavulanic acid with penicillin?**

This combination provides a synergistic effect. The clavulanic acid inhibits the activity of the beta lactamase enzymes and thus extends the action of the penicillin.

❑❑ **What inhibitors of beta lactamase are available for combining with penicillin?**

Clavulanic acid, sulbactam and tazobactam.

❏❏ Do the beta lactamase inhibitors have antibacterial activity?

No.

❏❏ What additional toxicity may be associated with the combinations of beta lactamase inhibitors with beta lactam antibiotics?

GI effects such as diarrhea.

❏❏ What is the advantage of amoxicillin over ampicillin?

Amoxicillin has better oral bioavailability.

❏❏ Are amoxicillin and ampicillin inactivated by penicillinase?

Yes.

❏❏ How do the cephalosporins differ from penicillins in their mechanism of action?

No difference, but they bind to different binding proteins.

❏❏ How are the cephalosporins usually classified?

By generation.

❏❏ How do the different generations of cephalosporins differ in their antibacterial spectrum?

First generation - Mainly gram positive organisms.
Second generation - Gram positive and a few gram negative organisms.
Third generation - Gram negative organisms.
Fourth generation - Gram negative with high degree of resistance to β-lactamase producing organisms.

❏❏ Which group of cephalosporins has the best penetration into the CNS?

Third generation.

❏❏ Does the dose of cephalosporins have to be modified in decreased renal function and why?

Yes, because these drugs are excreted mainly by the kidney?

❏❏ What is the major adverse effect associated with cephalosporin use?

Rashes and other hypersensitivity reactions.

❐❐ What other adverse effects are associated with the use of some of the cephalosporins?

Nephrotoxicity (mostly potential); Intolerance to alcohol; a positive Coomb's test; and hypoprothrombinemia.

❐❐ What is the drug of choice for the treatment of gonorrhea?

Ceftriaxone.

❐❐ What is the major use of the first generation cephalosporins?

As penicillin substitutes for gram positive infections when there is resistance or hypersensitivity to penicillin G.

❐❐ Which cephalosporins are considered as drugs of choice for the treatment of meningitis?

The third generation cephalosporins.

❐❐ Name a third generation cephalosporin with good activity against *Pseudomonas*?

Cefoperazone or ceftazidime.

❐❐ What types of infections are treated with the second generation cephalosporins?

Similar infections to those treated with first generation compounds plus several gram negative infections. Included among these are certain types of pneumonia, sinusitis, otitis and certain lower respiratory tract infections.

❐❐ What is the only presently approved fourth generation cephalosporin?

Cefepime.

❐❐ Which cephalosporin can be given orally, IM or IV?

Cephradine.

❐❐ What is a carbacephem and give an example?

A second generation cephalosporin with a carbon instead of an O or S in the thiazolidine ring e.g. loracarbef.

❐❐ What is the main advantage for using loracarbef?

Twice a day administration.

❐❐ What is imipenem?

A carbapenem antibiotic, similar to the beta-lactams but with a carbon in the 6 membered ring.

❒❒ What is the major advantage of imipenem?

It has the broadest antimicrobial spectrum of any beta-lactam antibiotic.

❒❒ Why must imipenem be administered with cilastatin?

Imipenem itself is hydrolyzed by a renal tubular enzyme so it is given along with cilastatin, an inhibitor of this enzyme.

❒❒ What type of infections is imipenem used to treat?

Infections caused by multi-drug resistant gram-negative organisms and complicated polymicrobial infections.

❒❒ What is the most serious toxicity associated with the use of imipenem?

Seizures.

❒❒ What is meropenem?

A more recently available carbapenem antibiotic.

❒❒ What are two advantages that meropenem has in comparison to imipenem?

It does not require coadministration with cilastatin and it has less likelihood of producing seizures than does imipenem.

❒❒ What is aztreonam?

A monobactam antibiotic.

❒❒ What is the major advantage for using aztreonam?

Patients who are allergic to penicillins or cephalosporins appear not to react to aztreonam.

❒❒ What group of antibiotics does aztreonam most closely resemble in terms of antimicrobial spectrum?

Aminoglycosides.

❒❒ What type of infections is aztreonam used for?

Its usefulness has not been completely defined but it is appropriately used for the treatment of moderate to severe aerobic gram negative infections.

❒❒ Name the commonly used macrolide antibiotics?

Erythromycin, clarithromycin and azithromycin.

❑❑ What ribosomal subunit do the macrolide antibiotics bind to?

50S.

❑❑ What other antibiotics bind to this subunit?

Clindamycin and chloramphenicol.

❑❑ Which step in protein synthesis is most likely inhibited by erythromycin?

Translocation.

❑❑ What are the advantages of the newer macrolide antibiotics over erythromycin?

Less GI irritation and better absorption.

❑❑ Erythromycin is the drug of choice or a co-drug of choice for the treatment of which type of infections?

Mycoplasma pneumoniae, legionnaires disease and chlamydial infections.

❑❑ What is the most serious toxicity associated with the use of erythromycin?

Cholestatic hepatitis.

❑❑ Which erythromycin preparation is cholestatic hepatitis most commonly associated with?

Erythromycin estolate (Ilosone).

❑❑ What is the major type of antibacterial activity associated with clindamycin?

Anaerobic organisms especially *Bacteroides fragilis*.

❑❑ What is the major therapeutic use of clindamycin?

Anaerobic infections, especially those caused by *Bacteroides fragilis*.

❑❑ What is the most serious toxicity associated with the use of clindamycin?

Pseudomembranous colitis (AAPC).

❑❑ How is AAPC caused?

By a toxin secreted by clindamycin resistant strains of *C.difficile*.

❑❑ What drugs are used to treat AAPC?

Vancomycin and metronidazole.

❏❏ How does vancomycin work?

Inhibition of cell wall biosynthesis at an earlier stage than that at which beta lactams act.

❏❏ How is vancomycin usually administered?

Parenterally (IV).

❏❏ What is the common toxicity associated with the use of vancomycin?

Red neck or red man syndrome.

❏❏ What are the two most serious toxicities associated with the use of vancomycin?

Ototoxicity and nephrotoxicity.

❏❏ Vancomycin is an important drug used for serious infections caused by which types of organisms?

Staphylococci and streptococci.

❏❏ What is teicoplanin?

A glycopeptide antibiotic that is very similar to vancomycin in mechanism of action and antibacterial spectrum.

❏❏ Name the aminoglycoside antibiotics?

Streptomycin, gentamicin, tobramycin, amikacin, netilmicin, kanamycin and neomycin.

❏❏ Aminoglycosides are mainly active against which group of bacteria?

Gram negative aerobes.

❏❏ Why are anaerobic bacteria not sensitive to aminoglycosides?

The aminoglycosides are poorly transported into anaerobes.

❏❏ What pharmacokinetic properties do all the aminoglycoside antibiotics share?

Poor absorption from the GI tract, poor penetration into the CNS and rapid renal excretion.

❏❏ What are the major toxicities associated with use of the aminoglycosides?

Ototoxicity, nephrotoxicity and neuromuscular blockade.

❏❏ What is the major cause of clinical resistance to the aminoglycoside antibiotics?

Increases in the enzymes metabolizing these drugs.

❑❑ **Aminoglycosides bind to which of the ribosomal subunits?**

30S.

❑❑ **What other antibiotics bind to this subunit?**

Tetracyclines.

❑❑ **What is the mechanism by which the aminoglycosides inhibit protein synthesis?**

Mainly by inhibition of protein synthesis initiation and miscoding.

❑❑ **Which aminoglycoside is used as a reserve drug for when there is resistance to the other aminoglycosides?**

Amikacin.

❑❑ **Which aminoglycosides are used in combination with the beta lactams for the treatment of serious pseudomonal infections?**

Gentamicin and tobramycin.

❑❑ **Which aminoglycoside is commonly used to treat T.B.**

Streptomycin.

❑❑ **What antibiotics are combined with aminoglycosides to treat enterococcal endocarditis?**

Beta-lactam antibiotics.

❑❑ **Why are the beta-lactams combined with the aminoglycosides?**

They are synergistic against certain bacteria (e.g. enterococci) in combination.

❑❑ **When beta lactams and aminoglycosides are used in combination they should not be mixed in the same solution, why is this?**

There is a physical incompatibility and you will precipitate out and inactivate the antibiotics.

❑❑ **What types of ototoxicity are associated with use of the aminoglycosides?**

Hearing loss and decreased vestibular function.

❑❑ **What is the mechanism for the ototoxicity caused by the aminoglycosides?**

The aminoglycosides accumulate in the organ of Corti and destroy the sensory hair cells located there.

❑❑ What factors can potentiate the ototoxicity associated with the use of the aminoglycosides?

Age of the patient, other ototoxic drugs (e.g. loop diuretics) and increased plasma levels of the antibiotics.

❑❑ What is the mechanism for the neuromuscular block produced by the aminoglycosides?

Inhibition of release of acetylcholine.

❑❑ What is the treatment for aminoglycoside induced neuromuscular blockade?

Anticholinesterase inhibitors and calcium.

❑❑ Which antibiotics can be used to treat anaerobic infections in the CNS?

Penicillin G, metronidazole and chloramphenicol.

❑❑ Describe the mechanism of action of metronidazole?

The anaerobic environment produces certain chemically active reduction products, which can disrupt DNA and inhibit nucleic acid synthesis.

❑❑ What are the therapeutic uses of metronidazole?

Anaerobic infections, trichomoniasis, amebiasis and giardiasis.

❑❑ What are the common adverse effects of metronidazole?

GI upset and some neurological toxicity (CNS effects and peripheral neuropathy).

❑❑ Why is metronidazole contraindicated in patients drinking alcohol?

It can produce an antabuse like reaction.

❑❑ The dose of metronidazole should be reduced in the presence of?

Decreased liver function.

❑❑ Name four antibiotics that should have their dose reduced with decreased liver function?

Erythromycin, chloramphenicol, metronidazole and clindamycin.

❑❑ Which two antibiotics have the broadest spectrum of antimicrobial activity?

Chloramphenicol and tetracyclines.

❑❑ What is the mechanism of action of chloramphenicol?

It binds to the 50S ribosomal subunit and reversibly inhibits protein synthesis most likely by inhibiting peptide bond formation.

❑❑ Which of the antibiotics that inhibit protein synthesis are bactericidal?

Aminoglycosides.

❑❑ Why are the aminoglycosides bactericidal?

The exact mechanism is not known but it may be related to their irreversible binding to the ribosomal subunit or to their ability to produce miscoding.

❑❑ What is the biochemical mechanism of resistance to chloramphenicol?

Increased acetyltransferase activity thus inactivating the drug.

❑❑ How is chloramphenicol metabolized?

Mainly by glucuronyltransferase.

❑❑ What is the gray baby syndrome?

Infants with their limited ability to metabolize chloramphenicol experience a syndrome, which includes as ashen gray cyanosis, which may be fatal.

❑❑ What type of toxicity limits the usefulness of chloramphenicol?

Idiosyncratic aplastic anemia.

❑❑ Is the idiosyncratic aplastic anemia dose related?

No, it is unrelated to dose.

❑❑ Does the idiosyncratic aplastic anemia occur during drug therapy?

No, it occurs after stopping therapy with the chloramphenicol.

❑❑ What other type of hematopoietic toxicity does chloramphenicol cause?

A dose related anemia.

❑❑ What is the mechanism of this dose related anemia?

Inhibition of mitochondrial protein synthesis.

❑❑ What types of infections is chloramphenicol useful for treating?

Typhoid fever, rickettsial diseases, bacterial meningitis, and anaerobic infections.

❒❒ Is chloramphenicol considered a first line drug?

No, it should only be used if a safer drug can't be used or is not tolerated by the patient.

❒❒ What precautions should be taken if chloramphenicol is used?

Periodic blood tests should be taken from the patient.

❒❒ Name three first generation tetracyclines?

Tetracycline, chlortetracycline and demeclocycline.

❒❒ What are the second-generation tetracyclines and what is their advantage?

Doxycycline and minocycline. They have a broader antimicrobial spectrum than the earlier generation of tetracyclines and have a greater lipophilicity.

❒❒ What is the mechanism of action of the tetracyclines?

They bind to the 30S ribosomal subunit and prevent access of aminoacyltRNA to the acceptor site on the mRNA -ribosome complex.

❒❒ How does resistance develop to the tetracyclines?

It most probably occurs as a result of increased efflux of the tetracycline out of the cell, which results from increased synthesis of a transporter protein.

❒❒ The half-life of which tetracycline remains unchanged in an anuric patient?

Doxycycline.

❒❒ Which tetracycline is most likely to cause dizziness and vertigo?

Minocycline.

❒❒ What compounds can interfere with tetracycline absorption and why?

Milk and dairy products, iron and other compounds with di- and tri- valent cations. These compounds chelate the tetracyclines and form insoluble complexes.

❒❒ Why are the tetracyclines contraindicated in young children.

They can cause discoloration of the teeth and can inhibit bone growth.

❒❒ What is the mechanism of the tetracyclines effect in bones and teeth?

Tetracyclines bind to calcium and then become deposited in the bones and teeth. Discoloration of the teeth is sometimes due to oxidation of the tetracycline-calcium complex.

❑❑ Why are tetracyclines contraindicated in pregnancy?

Tetracyclines have been known to cause hepatic necrosis, especially when given in large doses or in patients with preexisting liver impairment. Also they may stain the teeth of the fetus.

❑❑ What are some of the common toxicities of the tetracyclines?

GI upset, phototoxicity, renal toxicity, hepatic toxicity and effects on the teeth and bones.

❑❑ Tetracyclines are the treatment of choice for which diseases?

Rickettsial infections, chlamydial infections, lyme disease, mycoplasmal infections and chronic severe acne.

❑❑ Which antibiotics are used exclusively to treat UTIs?

Mandelamine, nalidixic acid, nitrofurantoin and fosfomycin.

❑❑ Why are these drugs used exclusively for UTIs?

High enough concentrations to be antibacterial are only obtained in the urinary tract and not in the systemic circulation.

❑❑ Nalidixic most closely resembles what group of antibiotics, structurally and mechanistically?

The quinolones.

❑❑ How does methenamine mandelate work?

It is first converted to formaldehyde after hydrolysis at an acid pH. Formaldehyde is the active antibacterial component.

❑❑ What are the major adverse effects associated with the use of nitrofurantoin?

Anorexia, nausea and vomiting are the major adverse effects associated with the use of nitrofurantoin.

❑❑ What is the mechanism of action of fosfomycin?

It inhibits an early stage in cell wall synthesis. It is an analog of phosphoenolpyruvate and inhibits the cytoplasmic enzyme enolpyruvate transferase which is the first step in the formation of UDP-N-acetylmuramic acid a cell wall precursor.

❑❑ How is fosfomycin used clinically?

In the U.S. only an oral preparation is available. It is approved for use as a single dose for treatment of uncomplicated lower UTIs in women.

❑❑ Amphotericin B belongs to which group of antifungal agents?

The polyene antifungals.

❑❑ Name another polyene used to treat fungal infections?

Nystatin.

❑❑ How is nystatin used clinically?

It is used topically to treat local candida infections.

❑❑ What is the mechanism of action of amphotericin B and the other polyenes?

It binds to ergosterol in the fungal cell membrane resulting in formation of pores that allow leakage of essential fungal nutrients. It also may have some effect on host cell macrophages thus boosting immunity.

❑❑ What unique structural characteristic of amphotericin and other polyenes account for this mechanism?

They have a significant number of both hydrophilic and hydrophobic groups in their structure.

❑❑ What types of fungi are sensitive to amphotericin B?

Several different kinds, including pathogenic yeasts, pathogenic yeast-like fungi, dimorphic fungi and molds or filamentous fungi.

❑❑ How was amphotericin traditionally administered?

As a colloidal dispersion in deoxycholate.

❑❑ What types of preparations are now available for Amphotericin B?

Lipid formulations.

❑❑ What are the advantages for the new lipid preparations of amphotericin B?

They alter the distribution of the amphotericin thus lessening the nephrotoxicity associated with it.

❑❑ How is amphotericin B used therapeutically?

It is mainly used to treat serious systemic fungal diseases; it is also used in select patients with profound neutropenia and fever unresponsive to broad-spectrum antibacterial agents.

❑❑ What is the most common adverse effect associated with the use of amphotericin B?

Nephrotoxicity occurs in about 80% of patients.

❑❑ What adverse effects are commonly associated with frequent infusion of amphotericin B?

Fever and chills and phlebitis at the site of the IV injection.

❑❑ Besides nephrotoxicity what types of dose-related toxicity are seen with amphotericin B?

A reversible normochromic, normocytic anemia and some neurotoxicity with intrathecal administration may occur.

❑❑ Describe the mechanism of action of flucytosine?

It is converted to 5-FU, which is phosphorylated to nucleotide forms and which then inhibits nucleic acid and protein synthesis in the fungi.

❑❑ What accounts for the selective toxicity of flucytosine (5-FC)?

The enzyme cytidine deaminase in fungi selectively converts 5-FC to 5-FU. Mammalian cells lack this enzyme.

❑❑ Is flucytosine a broad spectrum antifungal agent?

No, as it is active only against *Candida* and *Cryptococcus neoformans.* Most other fungi are resistant to the drug.

❑❑ Under what circumstances should the dose of 5-FC be reduced?

The dose should be altered in cases of decreased renal function.

❑❑ What are the principle adverse effects of flucytosine?

GI irritation, bone marrow depression and hepatic toxicity.

❑❑ What are the main therapeutic uses of flucytosine?

Cryptococcal and candida infections.

❑❑ Why is 5-FC usually given in combination with amphotericin B?

If fluorocytosine is used alone resistance occurs quickly.

❑❑ What are other advantages of combining 5-FC with amphotericin B?

You can decrease the dose of the amphotericin thus decreasing the toxicity and you also can get a synergistic effect from the two drugs.

❑❑ What are the azole antifungal drugs?

A group of broad spectrum orally effective antifungal agents with common structural features.

❑❑ **Which azoles are currently used systemically?**

Ketoconazole, fluconazole and itraconazole.

❑❑ **Describe the mechanism of action of the azole antifungal agents?**

They bind to cytochrome P-450 and inhibit the enzyme lanosterol 14-α-demethylase, thereby interrupting conversion of lanosterol to ergosterol which leads to accumulation of 14- α-methylsterols and depletion of ergosterol in the fungal cell wall. This in turn alters cell membrane properties and function and subsequently increases permeability and inhibits cell growth and replication.

❑❑ **What is the major difference between the older imidazoles and the newer triazoles?**

The newer triazoles are selective for fungal cytochrome P-450 while the older compounds bind to and inhibit both fungal and mammalian cell cytochrome P-450.

❑❑ **Ketoconazole absorption is dependent on what?**

A certain amount of gastric acidity.

❑❑ **What are the limitations for ketoconazole in the treatment of fungal disease?**

Little gets into the CNS so it is not very useful in meningitis, it is less effective in immunosuppressed patients and is not as effective in some of the more severe fungal infections.

❑❑ **What are the clinical uses of ketoconazole?**

A few systemic fungal infections and dermatophyte infections that are resistant to griseofulvin.

❑❑ **What adverse reactions are associated with the use of ketoconazole?**

GI intolerance, endocrine effects (decreased libido, oligospermia etc.) and hepatic toxicity.

❑❑ **What effect do antiulcer drugs have on the use of ketoconazole?**

By decreasing gastric acidity they inhibit the absorption of ketoconazole.

❑❑ **Why does ketoconazole interact with many other drugs?**

It inhibits the microsomal metabolism of several drugs (e.g. terfenadine).

❑❑ **How does the toxicity of itraconazole differ from ketoconazole?**

There is much less endocrine toxicity. GI distress is the most common effect seen.

❑❑ How is itraconazole used therapeutically?

For the treatment of serious systemic fungal diseases often associated with immunosuppression.

❑❑ What are the clinical uses of fluconazole?

Oral and IV treatment of cryptococcal meningitis and various forms of candidiasis.

❑❑ What are the most common adverse effects of itraconazole and fluconazole?

GI distress.

❑❑ Griseofulvin is used exclusively to treat what type of infections?

Dermatophytic infections (ringworm).

❑❑ How is griseofulvin administered?

It only works when given orally.

❑❑ What types of adverse effects are associated with griseofulvin use?

Headache, GI irritation, and rashes.

❑❑ How long must griseofulvin be given to be effective?

It depends on the location of the infection. Ringworm in the toenails or fingernails requires several months of treatment while that on the skin only a few days.

❑❑ Why are micronized preparations of griseofulvin used?

There is better absorption of the griseofulvin.

❑❑ What is the mechanism of action of griseofulvin?

At therapeutic doses it binds to tubulin and inhibits fungal mitosis.

❑❑ Why should periodic blood counts be taken after using griseofulvin?

It may suppress the bone marrow although this is rare.

❑❑ What types of drug-drug interactions can occur with griseofulvin?

It induces hepatic microsomal enzymes and thus could affect the metabolism of other drugs.

❑❑ Which drug is used to treat all types of T.B?

Isoniazid.

❑❑ **Why is combination therapy routine in the treatment of T.B.?**

To prevent the development of resistance.

❑❑ **Which drug should be used to prevent the development of active tuberculosis in a patient who recently converted to positive with a PPD test?**

INH.

❑❑ **What drug is added to antituberculosis regimens in order to kill the slow growing organisms in the macrophages and caseous lesions of tuberculosis?**

Pyrazinamide.

❑❑ **Why must you be careful as to which patients are given INH prophylactically?**

INH produces liver toxicity.

❑❑ **How does age effect the liver toxicity associated with the use of INH?**

Patients over 30 have an increased incidence.

❑❑ **What agent will prevent the neurotoxcity associated with the use of INH?**

Pyridoxine (Vitamin B6).

❑❑ **Name the five primary antituberculosis drugs?**

INH, rifampin, streptomycin, ethambutol and pyrazinamide.

❑❑ **Which is the only one of the first line anti-tuberculsis agents that must by given parenterally?**

Streptomycin.

❑❑ **When are the second line antiTB drugs used?**

When resistance develops or when therapy has been interrupted for another reason.

❑❑ **What is meant by the term directly observed therapy (DOT)?**

This refers to direct observation of the administration of antiTB drugs which increases compliance.

❑❑ **What is the standard antituberculosis therapy?**

INH plus rifampin plus pyrazinamide for 2 months then stop the pyrazinamide and continue therapy for an additional 4 months. In some cases four drugs are used initially and sometimes longer times of treatment are used.

❑❑ **Which are the additional first line drugs added to the regimen when a fourth drug is required?**

Ethambutol or streptomycin.

❑❑ **When are four drugs used to treat T.B.?**

When the incidence of resistance exceeds 4% in an area or the patients are recent immigrants who come from an area with known resistance or those with meningitis, AIDS or those with extensive pulmonary disease.

❑❑ **How should T.B. in AIDS patients be treated?**

Four drugs should be used and therapy should be extended for a year.

❑❑ **What is meant by intermittent therapy and when is it used?**

Twice a week or three times a week therapy with DOT. This improves compliance, but should be combined with directly observed therapy.

❑❑ **How is multiple drug resistant TB treated?**

Three or more drugs to which the organism is susceptible and therapy is continued for 12-24 months after the culture becomes negative.

❑❑ **What is the mechanism of action of isoniazid (INH)?**

It is now considered a prodrug and is converted to the active form by a catalase/peroxidase enzyme. The active form interferes with the biosynthesis of cell wall mycolic acids which results in disruption of the mycobacterial cell wall.

❑❑ **How does resistance develop to INH?**

It may involve loss of the gene for the catalase/peroxidase activity.

❑❑ **How is INH administered?**

Orally or parenterally, it shows similar bioequivalence when administered either way.

❑❑ **How is INH metabolized?**

Primarily by acetylation catalyzed by N-acetyltransferase.

❑❑ **How is this enzyme distributed throughout human populations?**

There are fast and slow acetylators of isoniazid and patients show genetic heterogeneity with regard to the rate of acetylation.

❑❑ **Does the acetylation status of a patient affect the therapeutic activity of INH?**

Usually not when INH is used daily.

❑❑ Does the acetylation status of a patient affect the toxicity of INH?

Slow acetylators show more peripheral neuropathy, while rapid acetylators show more liver toxicity.

❑❑ What is the mechanism of the liver toxicity associated with INH?

A hydrazine metabolite is the probable cause.

❑❑ What is the most common adverse effect associated with the use of INH?

Peripheral neuritis especially if pyridoxine is not given concurrently.

❑❑ Why does pyridoxine prevent the neurotoxicity associated with the use of INH?

INH causes pyridoxine deficiency by forming hydrazones that inhibit the conversion of pyridoxine to the active form pyridoxal phosphate.

❑❑ What potential drug-drug interactions may occur with INH?

It is a potential inhibitor of cytochrome P-450. It is also a potential inhibitor of monoamine and diamine oxidase.

❑❑ Why can INH increase the toxicity of acetaminophen?

Although usually an inhibitor of cytochrome P450 isozymes, INH can induce cytochrome p450 2E1 which metabolizes acetaminophen to a toxic metabolite.

❑❑ How is INH used clinically for TB?

It is the primary drug used for the treatment of active TB and is also used prophylactically.

❑❑ How is ethambutol used for the treatment of TB?

For the initial treatment in areas where there is a significant prevalence of drug resistance.

❑❑ What is the mechanism of action of ethambutol?

It probably inhibits arabinotransferase enzymes which are involved in the biosynthesis of the mycobacterial cell wall, but the exact mechanism is unknown and there is some evidence that RNA synthesis is also affected by ethambutol.

❑❑ What is the most common adverse reaction associated with the use of ethambutol?

Optic neuritis, manifested by decreased visual acuity, color blindness and decreased green color vision.

❑❑ Why is pyrazinamide only used for short course treatment of TB?

It becomes less effective after a couple of months, due to a decrease in the inflammatory response and an increase in the pH.

❑❑ What is the most common and serious side effect associated with pyrazinamide use?

Hepatotoxicity.

❑❑ How is rifampin used in the treatment of TB?

It is used for the initial treatment of TB, in the retreatment of TB and in intermittent therapy. It is also sometimes used in prophylactic therapy as an alternative to INH. and for the treatment of some atypical mycobacterial infections.

❑❑ What is the mechanism of action of rifampin?

It inhibits mycobacterial DNA-dependent RNA polymerase.

❑❑ How does resistance occur to rifampin?

By modification of the RNA polymerase beta subunit which decreases the binding affinity of the drug for its active site.

❑❑ How does the body excrete rifampin?

It is rapidly eliminated in the bile, followed by an enterohepatic recirculation. Eventually about 60% is excreted via the intestine.

❑❑ How is rifampin metabolized?

It is progressively deacetylated in the liver with the metabolite retaining full activity. It induces its own metabolism.

❑❑ What adverse effects are associated with the use of rifampin?

Gastrointestinal disturbances and hepatotoxicity.

❑❑ What additional toxicity is sometimes seen when rifampin is used in high dose intermittent therapy?

It produces several effects thought to have an immunological basis, including thrombocytopenia, hemolytic anemia, acute renal failure and the respiratory flu syndrome.

❑❑ What type of drug-drug interactions are associated with rifampin use?

Rifampin is a potent inducer of liver microsomal enzymes and may affect the metabolism of a variety of other drugs.

❏❏ Name five second line drugs used to treat T.B.?

Aminosalicylic acid, ethionamide, amikacin, kanamycin, capreomycin, cycloserine, ciprofloxacin, ofloxacin, clofazimine, rifapentine and rifabutin.

❏❏ When are the second line anti-T.B. drugs used?

When there is resistance or therapy has been stopped with the primary drugs for some other reason.

❏❏ What is the disadvantage of the second line drugs?

They have more toxic effects and less patient tolerability than the primary drugs.

❏❏ What is dapsone used for?

The long term treatment of leprosy.

❏❏ How does dapsone work?

Like the sulfonamides it inhibits folate synthesis.

❏❏ What adverse effects are associated with dapsone use?

Hemolysis, particularly if the patient has glucose-6-phosphate dehydrogenase deficiency, methemoglobinemia, GI intolerance, fever, pruritus and various rashes.

❏❏ What is clofazimine?

A phenazine dye that may be used as an alternative to dapsone. It is usually given for sulfone-resistant leprosy.

❏❏ What adverse effect is most prominent with clofazamine?

Skin discoloration ranging from red-brown to nearly black.

❏❏ Why was it more difficult to develop antiviral drugs than antibacterials?

Viruses are intracellular parasites that require the participation of the metabolic processes of the host cells. It is thus difficult to interfere with viral protein synthesis without also affecting cellular pathways.

❏❏ What are amantadine and rimantadine?

Cyclic amine compounds with activity vs RNA viruses.

❏❏ What is the antiviral activity of amantadine and rimantadine.

They inhibit the influenza A virus but have no activity vs influenza B.

❑❑ **What is mechanism of action of amantadine and rimantadine?**

They inhibit the M2 protein an ion channel. This effects viral uncoating and pH regulation in infected cells ultimately affecting viral replication.

❑❑ **What are the clinical uses of amantadine and rimantadine?**

They are used to prevent and treat influenza infections. For effective therapy they must be given within 48 hours of a flu infection.

❑❑ **How are amantadine and rimantadine handled by the body?**

Amantadine is primarily excreted in the urine, while rimantidine is extensively metabolized by the liver and doesn't depend on the kidney for elimination. Thus the dose of amantadine must be adjusted in decreased renal function.

❑❑ **What are the primary adverse effects of amantadine?**

Nausea and anorexia and CNS effects.

❑❑ **What are the major adverse effects of rimantadine?**

GI effects and rash, but less CNS effects than amantadine.

❑❑ **What groups of patients are especially susceptible to the CNS effects of amantadine?**

The elderly and those with decreased renal function.

❑❑ **What are the names of the two new antiinfluenza drugs that are specific inhibitors of viral neuraminidase.**

Zanamivir and oseltamivir.

❑❑ **What effect does inhibition of viral neuramindase have on the influenza infection?**

It stops the release of newly formed virus from the surface of infected cells and prevents viral spread across the mucus lining of the respiratory tract.

❑❑ **What antiviral activity do these two drugs have?**

They are both active vs. influenza A and B.

❑❑ **How are zanamivir and oseltamivir used clinically?**

To prevent and treat influenza infections although so far they have only been approved for treatment.

❑❑ **What is the major difference between zanamivir and oseltamivir?**

Zanamivir is given as a nasal spray, while oseltamivir can be given orally.

❑❑ **What are the adverse effects of zamamivir and oseltamivir?**

Nausea and vomiting.

❑❑ **Most of the antiherpes antiviral agents fit into what category of drugs?**

Purine or pyrimidine nucleosides.

❑❑ **What are the clinical uses of trifluridine?**

It is used topically for ocular herpes simplex keratitis infections.

❑❑ **Why can trifluridine only be used topically?**

If used systemically, it acts nonselectively on host cell DNA and can cause serious toxicity.

❑❑ **What is vidarabine?**

It is an adenosine analog, which is used as an antiviral drug.

❑❑ **What type of antiviral activity does vidarabine have?**

It is active against DNA viruses (mainly herpes viruses).

❑❑ **What is the mechanism of action of vidarabine?**

It is first phosphorylated to the corresponding nucleotides., then it acts as a competitive inhibitor of viral DNA polymerase and also is incorporated into DNA.

❑❑ **What is the limiting factor in the use of vidarabine?**

Its poor aqueous solubility means very large volumes would have to be injected.

❑❑ **What are the therapeutic uses of vidarabine?**

Herpes simplex keratitis, *Herpes simplex* encephalitis, *Herpes zoster*. It is presently not a first line drug for these diseases because acyclovir is safer and more effective.

❑❑ **What are the adverse reactions of vidarabine?**

GI effects are common, neurological toxicity can occur, several infusion related effects are seen including phlebitis, weakness, hypokalemia, rash, elevated liver enzymes, anemia, leukopenia and thrombocytopenia.

❑❑ **What adverse effects are seen when vidarabine is used topically in the eye?**

Lacrimation, burning, irritation, pain and photophobia.

❑❑ **Structurally what is acyclovir?**

An analog of guanosine or deoxyguanosine with an acyclic side chain.

❑❑ **What type of antiviral activity does acyclovir have?**

It has potent activity vs. the Herpes viruses.

❑❑ **What is the mechanism of action of acyclovir?**

It is phosphorylated to mono, di- and tri- phosphates. As the nucleotide it is an inhibitor of viral DNA polymerase and is incorporated into the growing DNA chain where it can act as a chain terminator due to the lack of the 3'- hydroxyl group.

❑❑ **Why is acyclovir more selective for viruses than other antiviral agents?**

It is selectively phosphorylated to the monophosphate form by viral thymidine kinase to the nucleotide form. It then selectively inhibits viral DNA polymerase.

❑❑ **How is acyclovir administered?**

It can be used orally, parenterally and topically.

❑❑ **What are the clinical uses of acyclovir?**

It is the drug of choice for a variety herpes infections (e.g. genital herpes, herpes keratitis). It is given I.V. for several serious Herpes simplex virus (HSV) infections or varicella zoster infections (VZV infections). It is also the treatment of choice for Herpes simplex encephalitis.

❑❑ **What is the most common adverse effect associated with the use of acyclovir?**

Renal toxicity.

❑❑ **What causes the renal toxicity associated with acyclovir?**

High urine levels of the drug cause crystalline nephropathy.

❑❑ **What factors contribute to the renal toxicity?**

Preexisting renal insufficiency, high doses of ACV and high plasma levels. Also rapid infusion, dehydration and inadequate urine flow.

❑❑ **Is the renal toxicity reversible?**

Yes, it usually resolves with drug cessation and volume expansion.

❑❑ **What other adverse effects are associated with the use of acyclovir?**

Neurotoxicity is uncommon and GI upset, headache and rash occur when it is given orally. There may also be lacrimation, itching, burning and pain when it is used in the eye.

❒❒ What is valacyclovir?

A prodrug of acyclovir that is rapidly converted to acyclovir after absorption. It has a mechanism of action identical to that of acylovir.

❒❒ What are the advantages of valacylovir?

It has excellent bioavailability. It results in serum levels orally similar to those achieved with IV administration of acyclovir and substantially higher serum levels than can be achieved with oral acyclovir.

❒❒ How is valacyclovir used therapeutically?

It has similar indications to that of acyclovir. It is also being studied for use in cytomegalovirus infections.

❒❒ What adverse effects are associated with the use of valacyclovir?

It is generally well tolerated, but a thrombotic thrombocyotpenic purpura/hemolytic anemia syndrome has been reported in some severely immunocompromised patients treated with high doses for prolonged periods. Hallucinations and confusion also may occur. Other adverse effects are similar to acyclovir.

❒❒ What is famcicolovir?

This is another prodrug. It is given orally and is converted to penciclovir, which is similar in structure to ganciclovir.

❒❒ What is the mechanism of action of famciclovir?

It has to be converted to the nucleotide form and then acts as an inhibitor of DNA polymerase. Unlike acyclovir it does not act as a DNA-chain terminator because of the presence of the 3' hydroxyl group; instead it is incorporated into the DNA molecule.

❒❒ What are the therapeutic uses of famciclovir?

It is used as an alternative to acyclovir. It has been effective in treating first episodes and recurrences of HSV and for its chronic suppression.

❒❒ What are the adverse effects of famciclovir?

It is generally well tolerated but headache, nausea and diarrhea have been reported.

❒❒ Is penciclovir itself used in therapy?

It is available as a topical cream. It may be helpful in treating recurrent orolabial herpes simplex virus infections in immunocompetent adults.

❑❑ How does ganciclovir differ from these other antiherpes nucleosides?

It is an analog of guanosine or deoxyguanosine with good activity against cytomegalovirus (CMV).

❑❑ Does ganciclovir work the same as acyclovir?

It is phosphorylated like acyclovir and the triphosphate also inhibits DNA polymerase. The triphosphate is a more avid inhibitor of viral than cellular DNA polymerase. Unlike acyclovir it may be incorporated directly into the enlarging DNA chain because it has a 3'-hydroxyl group.

❑❑ How is ganciclovir used clinically?

It is used to treat CMV infections, most commonly retinitis, colitis and esophagitis, in AIDS and other immunocompromised patients and to prevent and treat CMV disease in transplant patients.

❑❑ How is CMV disease treated when there is resistance to ganciclovir?

With foscarnet or cidofovir.

❑❑ What are the adverse effects of ganciclovir?

It is teratogenic, carcinogenic and mutagenic and causes aspermatogenesis in animals. Myelosuppression is the dose limiting toxicity. Granulocytopenia and thrombocytopenia are more common with the IV formulation and are usually reversible.

❑❑ What is foscarnet?

A pyrophosphate analog?

❑❑ What is the mechanism of action of foscarnet?

It is a noncompetitive inhibitor of viral DNA polymerase and reverse transcriptase but does not require prior phosphorylation to be active.

❑❑ How is foscarnet used clinically?

It is effective in treating CMV retinitis including progressive disease due to ganciclovir-resistant strains and in acyclovir resistant HSV or VZV infections.

❑❑ How does foscarnet compare to ganciclovir in its clinical use?

It is more expensive and generally less well tolerated than ganciclovir and requires controlled rates of infusion in large volumes of fluid.

❑❑ What adverse effects are associated with the use of foscarnet?

Renal dysfunction often develops with its use. Other effects are nausea, vomiting, anemia, fatigue, headache, genital ulceration and CNS disturbances. Hypo- and hypercalcemia, hypo- and hyperphosphatemia, hypokalemia and hypomagnesemia have also occurred.

❑❑ **What is cidofovir?**

It is an acyclic nucleoside phosphonate derivative.

❑❑ **How does cidofovir work?**

It inhibits DNA polymerase.

❑❑ **How is cidofovir used clinically?**

It is indicated for the treatment of CMV retinitis in patients with AIDS in whom treatment has failed or in those intolerant of therapy with ganciclovir or foscarnet.

❑❑ **What toxic effects are seen after the use of cidofovir?**

Severe nephrotoxicity is a dose-dependent major adverse effect.

❑❑ **What type of antiviral activity does ribavirin have?**

It is a broad-spectrum antiviral compound having activity against both DNA and RNA viruses.

❑❑ **What type of compound is ribavirin?**

It is a purine nucleoside (guanosine) analog.

❑❑ **What is the mechanism of action of ribavirin?**

Its mechanism is not well defined. Three possible mechanisms have been proposed all of which likely contribute to its antiviral activity. These include competitive inhibition of host enzymes resulting in reduced intracellular concentrations of GTP and decreased synthesis of DNA. Viral synthesis of protein is reduced by inhibition of the viral RNA polymerase complex. Messenger RNA formations are also inhibited. Ribavirin requires serial phosphorylation to the monophosphate, diphosphate and triphosphate forms by host cell kinases.

❑❑ **What are the therapeutic uses of ribavirin?**

Used as an aerosol it may decrease morbidity in some children hospitalized with respiratory syncytial virus (RSV), bronchiolitis and pneumonia. It has also been recently used in the treatment of hepatitis where combination treatment of hepatitis C with interferon alfa and oral ribavirin has produced higher sustained response rates than interferon or ribavirin alone.

❑❑ **What toxicities are associated with the use of ribavirin?**

Acute deterioration of respiratory function has been reported with ribavirin aerosol in infants and in adults with bronchospastic lung disease. Systemic ribavirin has been associated with hemolytic anemia. Ribavirin is teratogenic and embryotoxic in animals and is generally contraindicated in pregnancy.

❑❑ What are the interferons?

A group of host derived polypeptides with natural antiviral activity.

❑❑ What are the three kinds of interferons?

Interferon-alpha, beta, and gamma.

❑❑ What is the mechanism of action of the interferons?

They bind to specific cellular receptors. Through signal transduction pathways they induce synthesis of cellular enzymes that interfere with viral protein synthesis. They also stimulate the immune system.

❑❑ Which interferon is most useful commercially?

Interferon alfa.

❑❑ What are the therapeutic uses of interferon alfa?

It is used for treatment of hepatitis C, genital warts, Kaposi's sarcoma and various tumors.

❑❑ What are the adverse effects of interferon alfa?

I.M. or S.C. injection is commonly associated with an influenza-like syndrome, especially during the first week of therapy. High-dose or chronic therapy may be limited by bone marrow suppression, profound fatigue, myalgia and weight loss. Increased susceptibility to bacterial infections, psychiatric syndromes including depression, anxiety, emotional lability and agitation, increased aminotransferase activity, alopecia, hypo- or hyperthyroidism, tinnitus, reversible hearing loss, auto-antibody formation and possibly cardiotoxicity.

❑❑ What is the most common site of action of the antiAIDS drugs?

Inhibition of the reverse transcriptase enzyme in the human immunodeficiency virus (HIV).

❑❑ What are the nucleoside reverse transcriptase inhibitors (NRTIs)?

They were the first agents to be developed as anti AIDS drugs. They are similar to the natural nucleosides but differ from them by replacement of the hydroxy group in the 3' position by another group that is unable to form the 5' to 3' phosphodiester linkage essential for DNA elongation. They block reverse transcriptase activity by competing with the natural substrates and are incorporated into viral DNA to act as chain terminators in the synthesis of proviral DNA.

❏❏ What are the names of the nucleoside reverse transcriptase inhibitors available?

Zidovudine, stavudine, didanosine, zalcitabine, lamivudine and adefovir.

❏❏ What is the active form of the NRTIs?

They must first be intracellularly phosphorylated to their active 5' triphosphate forms by cellular kinases.

❏❏ How does resistance develop to the NRTIs?

The main mechanism for resistance is mutations in the *pol* gene that codes for the enzyme reverse transcriptase.

❏❏ What is zidovudine?

The first drug approved for treatment of AIDS. It is a thymidine analog and dideoxynucleoside in which a 3'-azido group replaces the 3'-hydroxyl group and has greater activity in replicating cells.

❏❏ What are some of the important pharmacokinetic properties of zidovudine?

It is well absorbed from the GI tract, it has good CNS penetration, and is metabolized in the liver by glucuronidation and is excreted by the kidneys. Dosage reduction is recommended in patients with severely impaired renal function.

❏❏ What is the major toxic effect of zidovudine?

Bone marrow suppression with resultant anemia, neutropenia or both. These are reversible upon discontinuation of the drug.

❏❏ What other toxicities are associated with zidovudine?

Myopathy and myositis are seen with prolonged use of zidovudine. Other effects are headache, nausea, vomiting, fatigue, malaise, insomnia and hyperpigmentation of the skin and nails.

❏❏ How is zidovudine used clinically?

In triple drug combinations for the treatment of AIDS, along with another NRTI and/or nonnucleoside reverse transcriptase inhibitor (NNRTI) and a protease inhibitor.

❏❏ What types of drug-drug interactions can be expected with zidovudine?

Other cytotoxic and myelosuppressive agents may potentiate the myelosuppressive properties of zidovudine. Ribavirin may inhibit the intracellular phosphorylation of zidovudine and thus decrease its antiretroviral activity.

❏❏ How does didanosine differ from zidovudine?

It is a synthetic purine nucleoside analog with hydrogen replacing the 3'-hydroxyl group. It has greater activity in resting peripheral blood mononuclear cells infected with HIV than in activated cells.

❑❑ How is didanosine administered?

Because it is unstable in acid conditions such as the gastric environment it is formulated with a buffer or antacids. It should be taken on an empty stomach.

❑❑ How is didanosine used clinically?

It is used primarily in combination with zidovudine or stavudine plus a protease inhibitor or NNRTI.

❑❑ What are the principal adverse effects of didanosine?

In contrast to zidovudine didanosine does not cause significant hematological effects. The major didanosine associated toxic effects are peripheral neuropathy and pancreatitis. Gastrointestinal complaints are also frequent. Because of nonoverlapping toxicities it is frequently used in combination with zidovudine.

❑❑ What is zalcitabine?

A synthetic pyrimidine nucleoside with activity against the AIDS virus. Similar to didanosine, zalcitabine has greater activity in resting peripheral blood mononuclear cells than in activated cells.

❑❑ How is zalcitabine used clinically?

Mainly in combination regimens with zidovudine and a protease inhibitor. It should not be combined with didanosine or stavudine because of overlapping toxicities.

❑❑ What is the major toxic effect of zalcitabine?

Peripheral neuropathy. Pancreatitis also occurs but less commonly than with zalcitabine.

❑❑ What is stavudine?

A synthetic thymidine analog that similar to zidovudine is preferentially phosphorylated and more potent in activated cells than in resting cells.

❑❑ What is the major toxic effect of stavudine?

Peripheral neuropathy, which is dose related and usually resolves with discontinuation of the drug or reduction of the dose.

❑❑ How is stavudine used clinically?

It is primarily used as an alternative to zidovudine in combination regimens among patients who cannot tolerate the hematological toxicity of zidovudine or who have progressive disease while on zidovudine containing regimens.

❑❑ How is lamivudine used clinically?

It is used mainly in combination with zidovudine or stavudine, plus a protease inhibitor or NNRTI. It is also approved for treatment of chronic hepatitis B.

❑❑ How does lamivudine work against the hepatitis virus?

It inhibits the DNA polymerase of hepatitis B virus after it is triphosphorylated.

❑❑ What are the major toxic effects of lamivudine?

GI intolerance, insomnia, headache, fatigue and skin rash.

❑❑ How does adefovir differ from the other NRTI's?

It is actually the first drug in a new class of nucleotide analog RT inhibitors that differ from nucleoside RT inhibitors in having an acyclic monophosphate component attached to the adenine base. This new structure results in antiviral activity against a broad range of viruses including HIV-1, HIV-2, hepatitis B virus and herpesviruses. It is also active against drug-resistant HIV strains.

❑❑ What are the clinical uses of adefovir?

It is used to treat AIDS where it may be especially useful in drug resistance, especially to zidovudine.

❑❑ What types of toxicity are associated with adefovir?

GI tract complaints, elevations in serum hepatic enzyme levels, weight loss, and delayed - onset nephrotoxicity, seen primarily as creatinine level elevations and hypophosphatemia.

❑❑ Which nonnucleoside reverse transcriptase inhibitors (NNRTIs) are clinically available?

Nevirapine, delavirdine and efavirenz.

❑❑ What is the mechanism of action of the NNRTIs?

They bind to the reverse transcriptase enzyme and bind to a unique site on the enzyme in a reversible and noncompetitive manner. The binding alters the ability of the enzyme to function. These drugs do not require cellular phosphorylation and are immediately active.

❑❑ What are the key pharmacokinetic properties of the NNRTIs?

Their oral bioavailability is good and their half-life is long which permits once daily administration for efavirenz or once- or twice- daily administration for nevirapine.

❑❑ What are the common adverse effects of the NNRTIs?

They produce a moderate rash especially at the beginning of therapy.

❒❒ What additional adverse effect is associated with efavirenz?

CNS symptoms (insomnia, somnolence and disturbing dreams) that usually disappears with time.

❒❒ How should the NNRTIs be used clinically?

In appropriate three-drug combinations for the treatment of AIDS. They should not be used alone or added to a failing regimen because resistance will rapidly develop.

❒❒ What types of drug-drug interactions will occur with the NNRTIs?

Nevirapine induces hepatic cytochrome P450 enzymes and delavirdine inhibits various P450 isoenzymes and thus the metabolism of other drugs given concurrently may be affected.

❒❒ What are the names of the protease inhibitors that are clinically available to treat AIDS?

Saquinavir, ritonavir, indinavir, nelfinavir and amprenavir.

❒❒ How do the protease inhibitors work as anti AIDS drugs?

They act in the later stages of the viral reproductive cycle and inhibit HIV replication in chronically infected cells and prevent the virus from infecting other cells. They inhibit the viral protease enzyme responsible for cleaving large, precursor polyproteins into smaller, functional proteins. This prevents formation of mature, infectious viral particles. They produce instead immature viruses incapable of infecting new cells. Combinations with reverse transcriptase inhibitors are synergistic.

❒❒ How does resistance develop to the protease inhibitors?

They arise from mutations in the protease genes.

❒❒ What are the key pharmacokinetic features of the protease inhibitors?

They have short half-lives and variable oral absorption.

❒❒ What are the adverse effects associated with the protease inhibitors?

All protease inhibitors can cause GI intolerance and increased aminotransferase activity. Metabolic disturbances such as insulin resistance and hyperlipidemia also may occur. These may preclude their lifelong use because of the potential risk of atherogenesis and thrombogenesis. These effects may result in changes in body shape such as lipodystrophy with facial fat wasting and add a psychological burden to therapy.

❒❒ What types of drug-drug interactions occur with the protease inhibitors?

Due to their extensive metabolism by the microsomal P450 liver enzymes specifically the CYP3A4 isoenzyme many drug interactions can occur. Therefore, medications that induce the activity of these isoenzymes (e.g. rifampin, phenobarbital and carbamazepine) can reduce protease inhibitor concentrations to subtherapeutic levels and result in the development of resistance. In addition, these drugs are themselves, to varying degrees inhibitors of this system which also leads to a number of interactions.

❑❑ **How are the protease inhibitors used clinically?**

In triple drug combinations with NRTI's for the treatment of AIDS.

❑❑ **What are the causal agents of malaria?**

Plasmodium falciparum, P.vivax, P.ovale and *P.malariae.*

❑❑ **What are the four major categories of antimalarial drugs?**

Blood schizonticides, tissue schizonticides, gametocytocides and sporontocides.

❑❑ **What are blood schizonticides?**

These are drugs that act rapidly on the erythrocytic stage of the malarial parasite to relieve clinical attacks. They make the person asymptomatic but often do not completely get rid of the parasite.

❑❑ **What drugs are considered effective blood schizonticides?**

Chloroquine, quinine, and mefloquine.

❑❑ **What is meant by the term tissue schizonticides?**

These drugs prevent relapse of malaria by acting on primary tissue forms in the liver.

❑❑ **Which drugs are tissue schizonticides?**

Primaquine.

❑❑ **What chemical group of compounds does chloroquine belong to?**

It is a 4-aminoquinolone.

❑❑ **Describe the mechanism of action of chloroquine?**

It reaches high concentrations in the food vacuole and interferes with heme polymerization and/or detoxification of the reactive oxygen species effectively killing the parasite with its own metabolic waste.

❑❑ **What is the mechanism of chloroquine resistance?**

It mainly results from decreased drug accumulation into the parasite digestive vacuole.

❑❑ **How is chloroquine administered?**

Oral or I.M. or S.C.

❑❑ **How is chloroquine used for malaria?**

It is used for acute attacks and prophylactically for chloroquine sensitive malaria.

❑❑ **What types of toxicity are associated with the use of chloroquine?**

When therapeutic or high doses are administered too rapidly parenterally there are primarily cardiovascular effects such as hypotension, vasodilation, EKG abnormalities etc. Oral chloroquine may cause GI upset, transient mild headache, urticaria, pruritus and visual disturbances. High doses and prolonged treatment with chloroquine can produce severe visual and cardiac reactions.

❑❑ **What type of compounds are quinine and quinidine?**

They are natural alkaloids isolated from the bark of the cinchona tree. Quinidine is an optical isomer of quinine.

❑❑ **How do quinine and quinidine work?**

Their mechanism of action is similar to chloroquine. They are not so extensively concentrated in the food vacuole and may act on alternative targets in the parasite.

❑❑ **How does resistance develop to quinine and quinidine?**

Resistance is probably due to increased efflux probably mediated through a homolog of P-glycoprotein.

❑❑ **How are quinine and quinidine administered?**

They are given by I.V infusion. They are rapidly acting compounds.

❑❑ **How are quinine and quinidine used in the treatment of malaria?**

They are used for chloroquine resistant and multi-drug resistant falciparum malaria. They are almost always used in conjunction with a sulfonamide or tetracycline. Quinidine is used in the U.S. for severe illness due to chloroquine and multi-drug resistant *P. falciparum.*

❑❑ **What are the toxic effects of quinine and quinidine?**

Cinchonism (tinnitus, headache, nausea, hearing and visual disturbances); hyperinsulinemia and severe hypoglycemia; severe hypotension when given too rapidly by i.v.; overdoses produce more severe symptoms including GI and C.V. disturbances. There may also be hemolysis in glucose-6-phosphate dehydrogenase deficient patients.

❑❑ **What is fansidar?**

A combination of sulfadoxine and pyrimethamine.

❑❑ **How is fansidar used in the treatment of malaria?**

It was formerly a first line agent but it is now occasionally used in conjunction with quinine or quinidine for serious disease caused by *P.falciparum*. It also has been used as a blood schizonticide to treat chloroquine resistant *P.falciparum* in a one-dose self-treatment in remote areas.

❑❑ What is the mechanism of action of fansidar?

The sulfa drug inhibits dihydropteroate synthetase and pyrimethamine is an inhibitor of dihydrofolate reductase. The two are synergistic in combination and result in a greater inhibition of folic acid synthesis than either alone.

❑❑ What is the toxicity of fansidar?

Antimalarial doses have little toxicity except occasional skin rashes and decreased hematopoiesis. High doses produce symptoms of folic acid deficiency (megaloblastic anemia.). The combination has produced severe and even fatal cutaneous reactions such as erythrema multiforme and Stevens Johnson syndrome..

❑❑ What group of compounds does primaquine belong to?

It is the only commonly employed member of the 8-aminoquinolones.

❑❑ What antimalarial drugs should be avoided in glucose-6-phosphate dehydrogenase (G-6-PDH) deficiency?

Primaquine, quinine, quinidine, fansidar, and chloroquine are all associated with hemolysis in these patients.

❑❑ What is the mechanism for the hemolysis produced when these drugs are given to patients with glucose-6-phosphate dehydrogenase deficiency?

In sensitive individuals G6PDH is low, and the cell consequently can't provide enough NADPH to keep up the levels of reduced glutathione in the presence of hemolyzing drugs. There is oxidative damage to erythrocyte membranes.

❑❑ What is the mechanism of action of primaquine?

It may interfere with electron transport in the malarial parasite, after conversion to electrophiles that act as oxidation-reduction mediators.

❑❑ How is primaquine used in the treatment of malaria?

It produces a radical cure when used in combination with chloroquine. Primaquine has an affect on the liver stages of the parasite and chloroquine or another blood schizonticide affects the blood stages.

❑❑ What are the adverse effects of primaquine?

GI upset, nausea, headache are most common. Larger doses may cause hemolytic anemia, cyanosis and leukocytosis.

❑❑ What is the mechanism of action of mefloquine?

It is similar to quinine in many aspects.

❑❑ What is the clinical use of mefloquine in malaria?

It is a blood schizonticide used only for the treatment and prophylaxis of chloroquine-resistant and multi-drug resistant *P.falciparum* malaria.

❑❑ What adverse effects are associated with the use of mefloquine?

GI upset is common, CNS toxicity is seen in half of the people who take it. Severe neuropsychiatric reactions are rare but possible.

❑❑ What is artemisinin and its derivatives?

An extract of a Chinese plant with antimalarial activity.

❑❑ How is artemisinin and its derivatives used in malaria treatment?

It is especially useful to treat chloroquine resistant *P.falciparum* malaria.

❑❑ How is doxycycline used in the treatment of malaria?

It is used for the treatment and prophylaxis in regions where multi-drug resistance is common.

❑❑ What types of drugs are used to treat amebiasis?

Luminal amebicides are used for the intestinal forms of the parasite and can be used to treat both asymptomatic patients or those with mild intestinal infections. The invasive form of amebiasis is treated with systemic amebicides and then we have drugs that work against both intestinal and invasive forms of the parasite.

❑❑ What drugs are used to treat the asymptomatic cyst passer and mild intestinal infections?

Iodoquinol and paromomycin are the treatments of choice. Both are luminal amebicides.

❑❑ What types of toxicity are associated with the use of iodoquinol and paromomycin?

Usually absorption is little so only GI upset and diarrhea occurs. Iodoquinol can produce subacute myelooptic neuropathy although it is rare.

❑❑ What drug is used for the treatment of all symptomatic cases of amebiasis including those with liver involvement?

Metronidazole.

❑❑ Why is a luminal amebicide given with metronidazole?

Absorption is higher up in the intestine and thus metronidazole is not effective against the luminal organisms.

❑❑ What is the treatment of choice for trichomoniasis and giardiasis?

Metronidazole.

❑❑ Which benzimidazoles are used to treat helminth infections?

Mebendazole, thiabendazole and albendazole.

❑❑ What is the mechanism of action of the benzimidazole anthelminthic drugs?

Inhibition of microtubule polymerization by binding to tubulin.

❑❑ Why is mebendazole very useful for the treatment of intestinal parasite infections?

Its absorption after oral administration is poor and erratic.

❑❑ What are the main therapeutic uses of mebendazole?

It is a broad spectrum anthelmintic. It is highly effective against GI nematode infections including roundworms, hookworm, whipworm and pinworm. It is particularly valuable for mixed infections.

❑❑ What are the therapeutic uses of thiabendazole?

It is the drug of choice for "cutaneous larval migrans" caused by the larvae of the dog hookworm. It is also an alternative for infestations with *Strongyloides stercoralis* a nematode infection.

❑❑ What toxic effects are associated with thiabendazole use?

Anorexia, nausea, vomiting and diarrhea are frequent. Less frequent are certain CNS effects such as dizziness, weariness, hallucinations, drowsiness, giddiness and headaches. Occasionally there might be fever and some rashes. Hepatotoxicity is a potential effect.

❑❑ What are the therapeutic uses for albendazole?

It has a broad range of activity vs. many nematodes and cestodes. It is also the treatment of choice for cystic hydatid disease and for neurocysticercosis.

❑❑ Which anthelmintic agent is the drug of choice for all forms of schistosomiasis.

Praziquantel.

❑❑ What is the mechanism of action of praziquantel?

It interferes with calcium homeostasis. There is increased muscular activity followed by contraction and spastic paralysis at low doses. The affected worms detach from host tissues and may shift from the mesenteric veins to the liver or are expelled from the body. At higher concentrations there is tegument damage and activation of host defense mechanisms that may result in destruction of the worm.

❑❑ What adverse effects are seen with praziquantel?

Overall it is well tolerated. There is abdominal discomfort, particularly pain and nausea, headache, dizziness and drowsiness.

❑❑ What is the mechanism of action of ivermectin?

Potentiation and direct activation or both of glutamate gated chloride channels found only in invertebrates. This results in an influx of negatively charged ions.

❑❑ What are the therapeutic uses of ivermectin?

Onchocerciasis, lymphatic filariasis and infections with intestinal nematodes.

❑❑ What type of toxicity is associated with the use of ivermectin?

A Mazzotti like reaction from the dying microfilariae. This is an allergic-type reaction.

❑❑ What are the clinical uses of pyrantel pamoate.

Pinworm, roundworm and hookworm infections.

❑❑ How does pyrantel work?

It produces a depolarizing neuromuscular block in the worms. There is a marked persistent activation of nicotinic receptors, which results in spastic paralysis of the worm.

❑❑ What are the adverse effects associated with the use of pyrantel?

It is given orally and toxic effects are seen only with very large doses. There are transient and mild GI symptoms occasionally as well as headache, dizziness, rash and fever.

❑❑ What is meant by an opportunistic infection?

They are infections occurring in immunocompromised patients.

❑❑ Why are they more difficult to treat in AIDS patients?

In AIDS patients these diseases have a different pathophysiology and may require a different therapeutic approach.

❑❑ What is the most common opportunistic infection that occurs in patients having AIDS?

PCP (*Pneumocystis carinii* pneumonia).

❑❑ **What is the treatment of choice for PCP?**

Cotrimoxazole (sulfamethoxazole/trimethoprim).

❑❑ **What is the drug of choice for preventing PCP?**

Cotrimoxazole.

❑❑ **What is the major alternative drug for both treatment and prevention of PCP?**

Pentamidine.

❑❑ **Why is cotrimoxazole preferred to pentamidine for the treatment of PCP?**

It is equally effective but produces less toxicity than pentamidine.

❑❑ **How is pentamidine usually given for prophylaxis?**

It is given as an aerosol.

❑❑ **Why is pentamidine given as an aerosol?**

There is less toxicity.

❑❑ **What type of toxicity is usually associated with cotrimoxazole when it is used to treat PCP in AIDS patients?**

Rash, nausea, fever and leukopenia are frequent.

❑❑ **What types of toxic effects are usually associated with pentamidine when it is used to treat or prevent PCP in AIDS patients?**

Pain at the site of I.M. injection, along with erythema and formation of sterile abscesses. I.V. administration is associated with breathlessness, tachycardia, dizziness or fainting, headache or vomiting. Rapid I.V. use is associated with hypotension. Other serious toxicities are nephrotoxicity, pancreatitis, hypoglycemia, diabetes, leukopenia, cardiac arrhythmias and prolonged orthostatic hypotension.

❑❑ **What is the standard therapy for treating toxoplasmosis in AIDS patients?**

Pyrimethamine plus sulfadiazine.

❑❑ **Why is folinic acid usually given concurrently with pyrimethamine plus sulfadiazine therapy?**

To attentuate the leukopenia and thrombocytopenia due to the pyrimethamine.

❑❑ **How does pyrimethamine work?**

It is a selective inhibitor of parasitic dihydrofolate reductase.

❑❑ What toxicity is commonly associated with the use of pyrimethamine?

Megaloblastic anemia.

❑❑ What is the standard therapy for tuberculosis in AIDS patients?

Nine month therapy with INH, rifampin or rifabutin, pyrazinamide plus ethambutol or streptomycin.

❑❑ Why is rifabutin preferred if the patient is taking protease inhibitors or NNRTIs?

Rifabutin is a less potent inducer of microsomal enzymes and thus the chances of drug interactions are less.

❑❑ Which is the drug of choice for preventing *Mycobacterium avium* complex (MAC)?

Clarithromycin or azithromycin.

❑❑ What drugs are used for the treatment of MAC?

Rifampin, rifabutin, ethambutol, ciprofloxacin and azithromycin or clarithromycin.

❑❑ What additional adverse effect may occur when the macrolides are used in the treatment of MAC compared to other patients?

Ototoxicity (tinnitus, dizziness and reversible hearing loss).

❑❑ How does rifabutin work?

The same as rifampin, inhibition of DNA dependent RNA polymerase.

❑❑ How does the activity of rifabutin vs MAC compare to rifampin?

Rifabutin is more active.

❑❑ Compared to rifampin what additional toxicity is of concern when using rifabutin?

Uveitis.

❑❑ Does rifabutin affect the activity of zidovudine?

Yes, it decreases its plasma levels.

CANCER CHEMOTHERAPY AND IMMUNOPHARMACOLOGY

CANCER CHEMOTHERAPY

❑❑ **Which phase of the cell cycle is most resistant to chemotherapeutic agents?**

$G_{0.}$

❑❑ **Which phase of the cell cycle is most sensitive to anticancer drugs?**

S.

❑❑ **Which group of drugs must be first converted to nucleotides before they are active as anticancer agents?**

Purine and pyrimidine antimetabolites.

❑❑ **Anticancer drugs are most effective against what type of tumors?**

Rapidly growing tumors.

❑❑ **Do anticancer drugs kill a constant number of tumor cells?**

No, they kill a constant fraction of tumor cells.

❑❑ **What is meant by the term adjuvant therapy?**

The use of chemotherapy following surgery or radiation.

❑❑ **What is the rationale for adjuvant therapy?**

The surgery or radiation removes most of the tumor leaving a small rapidly growing tumor or its metastases. These smaller tumors are more sensitive to the subsequent chemotherapy.

❑❑ **What is meant by the term neoadjuvant therapy?**

The use of chemotherapy first and then surgery.

❑❑ **What is meant by multidrug resistance (MDR)?**

Cross resistance to several unrelated anticancer compounds.

❒❒ What are the biochemical consequences of MDR?

More drug is actively pumped out of the cell resulting in a decreased effect.

❒❒ Multidrug resistance is most likely the result of amplification of which gene?

MDR1 which codes for a transport protein p170.

❒❒ What are the advantages of combination chemotherapy in cancer treatment?

It may decrease the likelihood of resistance developing and there may be synergistic effects.

❒❒ What types of drugs are used in combination chemotherapy?

Drugs with different mechanisms of action, drugs with different toxicities (especially drugs which are non-myelosuppressive) and drugs which alone have some anticancer activity.

❒❒ Name four nitrogen mustards.

Mechlorethamine, chlorambucil, cyclophosphamide and melphalan.

❒❒ Explain the mechanism of action of the nitrogen mustard agents?

They form a carbonium ion, which then interacts with nucleophiles like those present in nucleic acids and proteins. Interaction with the guanine in DNA is a key site of action. They are cytotoxic mainly as a result of forming cross-links in DNA.

❒❒ What is MOPP and what is it used for?

It is an acronym for the combination treatment for Hodgkins disease (Mechlorethamine, Oncovin, Prednisone and Procarbazine).

❒❒ Which is the most versatile of the alkylating agents?

Cyclophosphamide.

❒❒ How is cyclophosphamide activated?

By liver microsomal enzymes to phosphoramide mustard, which is believed to be the active anticancer metabolite and acrolein believed to be the cause of the bladder toxicity associated with cyclophosphamide

❒❒ How do the nitrosoureas differ from other alkylating agents?

The main difference is that they are more lipid soluble.

❒❒ How are the nitrosoureas activated?

Nonenzymatically to form a carbonium ion and an isothiocyanate compound.

❑❑ How is nitrogen mustard (mechlorethamine) administered and why?

Through a running IV infusion. If not given that way it could be accidentally extravasated and once on ther skin can cause blistering.

❑❑ What is the treatment of choice for chronic lymphocytic leukemia?

Chlorambucil.

❑❑ What is the dose-limiting toxicity of the alkylating agents?

Bone marrow suppression.

❑❑ What is the major therapeutic use of busulfan?

Treatment of chronic myelogenous leukemia.

❑❑ Name three nitrosoureas available for therapeutic use.

Carmustine (BCNU), lomustine(CCNU), and semustine (methylCCNU).

❑❑ Which alkylating agents are associated with the production of hemorrhagic cystitis?

Cyclophosphamide and iphosphamide.

❑❑ Which metabolite of cyclophosphamide is most probably the cause of the hemorrhagic cystitis associated with cyclophosphamide use.

Acrolein.

❑❑ How can the hemorrhagic cystitis produced by iphosphamide and cyclophosphamide can be reduced ?

Administration of MESNA and adequate hydration of the patient. MESNA is a sulfhydryl compound which interacts with the alkylating agents before they interact with tissue.

❑❑ The mechanism of action of cisplatin most closely resembles that of which group of anticancer compounds?

Alkylating agents.

❑❑ Cisplatin is useful to treat what types of cancer?

Testicular cancer, bladder cancer, head and neck cancer, ovarian cancer and lung cancer.

❑❑ What is the dose limiting toxicity of cisplatin?

Nephrotoxicity.

❑❑ What is the dose limiting toxicity of carboplatin?

Bone marrow depression.

❑❑ Which type of cancer is dacarbazine is used to treat?

Malignant melanoma.

❑❑ What type of acute toxicity is cisplatin associated with?

Nausea and vomiting.

❑❑ What is the advantage of carboplatin over cisplatin?

It has less toxicity. It has a low potential for ototoxicity, nephrotoxicity and peripheral neuropathy.

❑❑ How would you describe the mechanism of action of actinomycin D.

It intercalates into DNA and blocks DNA directed RNA synthesis.

❑❑ Which anticancer drugs develop resistance as result of amplification of the multi-drug resistance gene (MDR)?

Actinomycin, doxorubicin, daunorubicin, vinca alkaloids and taxol compounds.

❑❑ Which anticancer drugs should be administered through a running IV infusion?

Actinomycin D, vinca alkaloids, anthracyclines and mechlorethamine.

❑❑ Actinomycin D is very effective in the treatment of which types of tumors?

Pediatric solid tumors and choriocarcinoma which is methotrexate resistant.

❑❑ What is the dose limiting toxicity of Actinomycin D?

Bone marrow suppression.

❑❑ What is the radiation recall effect?

An additive effect on the skin as a result of a drug like actinomycin and previous radiation treatment.

❑❑ What is the somewhat unique rate limiting toxicity of the anthracycline antibiotics?

Cardiotoxicity.

❑❑ What other toxic effects are associated with the use of the anthracycline drugs?

Bone marrow suppression, stomatitis, GI effects, alopecia and the radiation recall effect.

❑❑ What is the likely mechanism of the cardiotoxicity associated with the use of the anthracylcines?

Free radical production.

❑❑ How can this toxicity be prevented or treated?

Keep the dose below 500 mg/M^2 or use free radical scavengers like dexrezoxane.

❑❑ How are doxorubicin and daunorubicin handled by the body?

Hepatic metabolism followed by biliary excretion.

❑❑ How do the therapeutic uses of doxorubicin and daunorubicin differ?

Daunorubicin is used mainly to induce remission in acute leukemias while doxorubicin is a very valuable drug in the treatemnt of solid tumors like breast cancer.

❑❑ Describe the mechanism of action of the anthracycline antibiotics?

Intercalation into DNA, free radical production with DNA strand breakage and inhibition of topoisomerase II. The current thinking is that inhibition of topoisomerase is the most important effect of these drugs.

❑❑ Describe how resistance develops to the anthracycline antibiotics?

Predominantly through enhanced efflux as a result of increased expression of the MDR gene.

❑❑ What is the advantage of the anthracenedione drug mitoxanthone over the anthracyclines?

It has less cardiotoxicity.

❑❑ What are etoposide and its close relative teniposide?

They are semisynthetic glycosidic derivatives of podophyllotoxin obtained from the roots and rhizomes of the Mayapple plant.

❑❑ Explain the mechanism of action of etoposide and teniposide?

They inhibit toposisomerase II with accompanying breaks in DNA.

❑❑ How does resistance develop to these drugs?

Amplification of the MDR gene and decreased expression of toposomerase II.

❑❑ How are etoposide and teniposide administered?

IV, as their absorption is variable with oral administration.

❏❏ Describe how etoposide and teniposide are used clinically?

Their major uses are for the treatment of testicular tumors and small cell lung carcinomas in combination with other drugs. Other uses include Hodgkins and Non Hodgkins lymphomas and teniposide is sometimes used for refractory ALL.

❏❏ What is the dose limiting toxicity of etoposide and teniposide?

Bone marrow suppression.

❏❏ Name the drugs that inhibit topoisomerase I.

Camptothecin derivatives like topotecan and irinotecan.

❏❏ What is the function of topoisomerase I?

It induces single strand breaks in supercoiled DNA and once the torsional strain is released the enzyme reseals the break and disassociates from the DNA.

❏❏ How does topoisomerase I differ from topoisomerase II?

It is not cell cycle specific like topo II and its function is independent of ATP.

❏❏ What are the topoisomerase I inhibitors used for therapeutically?

To treat a variety of solid tumors.

❏❏ What are the dose limiting toxicities of topotecan and its derivatives?

Bone marrow suppression.

❏❏ What is bleomycin?

A mixture of glycopeptides with anticancer activity vs. squamous cell tumors.

❏❏ What accounts for the anticancer action of bleomycin?

It causes fragmentation of the DNA.The drug binds to iron and to DNA by intercalation. Oxygen free radicals are produced which cleave the DNA.

❏❏ How does resistance develop to bleomycin?

High levels of bleomycin hydrolase metabolize the bleomycin to inactive compounds.

❏❏ How is bleomycin administered?

Parenterally.

❒❒ What group of tumors is bleomycin especially active against?

Squamous cell carcinomas.

❒❒ To treat testicular tumors bleomycin is combined with which other anticancer drugs?

Cisplatin and vinblastine.

❒❒ Why is bleomycin frequently used in combination chemotherapy?

It is non bone marrow suppressive while most anticancer agents are bone marrow suppressive.

❒❒ What is the most common toxicity associated with the use of bleomycin?

Toxicity to the skin and mucus membranes.

❒❒ What is the dose limiting toxcity of bleomycin?

Pulmonary toxicity.

❒❒ Why is bleomycin especially toxic to the skin and mucus membranes?

These organs have low levels of bleomycin hydrolase.

❒❒ What is meant by the term antimetabolite?

An antimetabolite is a drug that resembles the natural metabolite in structure but has enough differences so as to interfere with the metabolism of that metabolite.

❒❒ What are the three groups of antimetabolites used in cancer chemotherapy?

Folate antagonists, purine antimetabolites and pyrimidine antimetabolites.

❒❒ How do antimetabolites kill tumor cells?

The mechanism of death is not completely understood but it is believed to be related to unbalanced growth whereby DNA synthesis is inhibited but not RNA and protein synthesis.

❒❒ Are antimetabolites selective for tumor cells?

No, they inhibit the growth of most rapidly proliferating cells in the body (e.g. bone marrow, GI tract etc.).

❒❒ What is the basis for the selective toxicity of methotrexate?

It binds to and inhibits tumor cell dihydrofolate reductase several hundred fold greater than the normal cell enzyme.

❑❑ What is the mechanism of action of methotrexate?

Inhibition of dihydrofolate reductase. This in turn results in inhibition of thymidylate synthetase and DNA synthesis through folate depletion.

❑❑ What phase of the cell cycle do the antifolates work at?

S phase.

❑❑ How does resistance develop to methotrexate?

Probably through multiple mechanisms including decreased uptake, amplification of the reductase gene and a decreased ability to form methotrexate polyglutamates inside the cell.

❑❑ How is methotrexate administered?

Orally (chronic or intermittent); intermittent or high dose IV and intrathecally.

❑❑ What property of methotrexate results in it being potentially involved in many drug interactions?

Methotrexate binds to plasma proteins to the extent of around 50% so it can displace other drugs from these binding sites or it can be displaced itself by other drugs.

❑❑ What are the principal therapeutic uses of methotrexate in cancer chemotherapy?

It is used to treat gestational choriocarcinoma, ALL in children, to prevent CNS relapse of ALL, in combination therapy for breast cancer and to treate osteogenic cancer (high dose rescue therapy).

❑❑ What compound reverses all of the toxic effects of methotrexate except the neurotoxicity?

Leucovorin (folinic acid, citrovorum factor).

❑❑ What is the earliest sign of methotrexate toxicity?

Mucositis (inflammation of the gums).

❑❑ What is the most serious form of methotrexate toxicity?

Bone marrow suppression.

❑❑ What is meant by high dose methotrexate therapy?

High doses of methotrexate plus leucovorin.

❑❑ What is the rationale behind high dose methotrexate therapy?

You give high doses to kill more tumor cells and selectively rescue normal cells with the presence of leucovorin.

❑❑ What are the clinical uses for high dose methotrexate therapy?

Osteogenic sarcoma, prevention of leukemic meningitis, and non-Hodgkins lymphoma.

❑❑ What additional toxicities may be associated with the use of high dose methotrexate therapy?

Renal toxicity due to precipitation of the 7-hydroxy metabolite.

❑❑ Which purine antimetabolites have been commonly used in cancer chemotherapy?

6-mercaptopurine and thioguanine. Recently fludaribine and cladribine have been introduced into therapy.

❑❑ What is the active form of the purine antimetabolites?

The nucleotide or triphosphate form.

❑❑ What enzyme catalyzes formation of the nucleotide from the thiopurines?

Phosphoribosyltransferase.

❑❑ What is the mechanism of action of the purine antimetabolites?

The exact mechanism is unknown, but it probably involves a combination of effects including inhibition of the first enzyme in *de novo* purine synthesis, inhibition of nucleotide interconversion and incorporation of the triphosphates into nucleic acids.

❑❑ How does resistance develop to the purine antimetabolites?

In experimental tumors it probably results from a lack of or an altered phosphoribosyltransferase enzyme. In human tumors increased alkaline phosphatase and increased catabolism is probably a major cause.

❑❑ If a person is resistant to one purine antimetabolite, can another one be used?

No, because there is cross resistance between the different purine antimetabolites.

❑❑ How are 6-MP and 6-TG administered?

Orally, even though oral absorption is often slow and variable.

❑❑ How is 6-MP metabolized?

It is either methylated or oxidized to thiouric acid.

❒❒ What enzyme oxidizes 6-MP to thiouric acid?

Xanthine oxidase.

❒❒ What are the therapeutic uses of 6-MP?

Acute lymphocytic leukemia (ALL) for maintenance therapy.

❒❒ What are the therapeutic uses of 6-TG?

Acute myelogenous leukemia (AML) (usually in combination with ARA-C and daunomycin) to induce remissions.

❒❒ What toxicities are associated with the use of the purine antimetabolites?

Bone marrow suppression is rate limiting. Nausea and vomiting also occur and 6-MP produces hepatotoxicity.

❒❒ What is the purpose of combining 6-MP with allopurinol?

The allopurinol inhibits the metabolism of the purine increasing its effectiveness.

❒❒ What is the negative side of combining 6-MP with allopurinol?

The toxicity is also increased.

❒❒ Why is allopurinol sometimes added to anticancer therapy?

To prevent the hyperuricemia and hyperuricosuria associated with killing large numbers of cells quickly.

❒❒ Name the fluoropyrimidine analogs used in cancer chemotherapy?

5-fluorouracil (5-FU) and fluorodeoxyuridine (FdUrd).

❒❒ What is the active form of the anticancer fluoropyrimidines?

The nucleotide form.

❒❒ What is the mechanism of action of 5-FU?

Conversion to FdUMP followed by inhibition of thymidylate synthetase. In addition 5-FU after phosphorylation is incorporated into both DNA and RNA. This may result in DNA strand breakage and inhibition of certain RNA functions.

❒❒ What are the therapeutic uses of the fluoropyrimidines?

Solid tumors such as breast cancer, gastrointestinal and gynecologic tumors.

❒❒ How is 5-FU used topically?

For the treatment of basal cell carcinomas and premalignant keratoses.

❑❑ **What are the major toxicities of FU?**

Bone marrow suppression when given by IV bolus and GI when given by continuous infusion.

❑❑ **What is cytosar?**

Cytosine arabinoside (Ara-C), a deoxycytidine analog.

❑❑ **How does cytosine arabinoside work?**

It is converted to the nucleotide triphosphate analog. This is followed by inhibition of DNA synthesis as a result of inhibition of DNA polymerase and inhibition of DNA chain elongation.

❑❑ **How is cytosine arabinoside used therapeutically?**

It is used to induce remission of leukemias in children and adults usually in combination with 6-TG and one of the anthracyclines.

❑❑ **What is the dose limiting toxicity of cytosine arabinoside?**

Bone marrow suppression.

❑❑ **What is the "cerebellar syndrome"?**

It refers to the neurotoxicity associated with high dose cytosine arabinoside therapy.

❑❑ **What is gemcitabine?**

It is a deoxycytidine analog used as an anticancer agent.

❑❑ **How is gemcitabine used clinically?**

It has broad spectrum antitumor activity particularly in tumor types chemoresistant to other chemotherapy.

❑❑ **Where are the vinca alkaloids obtained from?**

The leaves of the periwinkle plant.

❑❑ **What is the mechanism of action of the vinca alkaloids?**

They bind to tubulin and prevent microtubules from aggregating.

❑❑ **What phase of the cell cycle are the vinca alkaloids active against?**

Mitosis.

❒❒ **What causes resistance to the vinca alkaloids?**

They are part of the MDR complex. Amplification of the gp170 results in increased efflux of the vinca alkaloids out of the cell.

❒❒ **How are the vinca alkaloids administered therapeutically?**

They are given by IV infusion, in a rapidly flowing IV infusion to prevent skin damage if extravasated.

❒❒ **How is vincristine used therapeutically?**

It is used to induce remission in acute lymphocytic leukemia and to treat Hodgkins lymphoma in combination with other drugs.

❒❒ **How is vinblastine used therapeutically?**

It is effective in the treatment of Hodgkins disease and non-Hodgkins lymphoma and most importantly metastatic testicular tumors along with bleomycin and cisplatin.

❒❒ **What is the difference in toxicity between vincristine and vinblastine?**

Vincristine produces mostly neurological toxicities such as peripheral neuropathy while vinblastine produces mostly bone marrow suppression.

❒❒ **What is the mechanism of action of the taxol derivatives?**

The taxols cause stabilization of the microtubules and formation of abnormal bundles of microtubules.

❒❒ **What are the therapeutic uses of the taxols.**

They are used to treat several solid tumors, such as ovarian, lung and breast cancer.

❒❒ **What are the major toxic effects of the taxols?**

Bone marrow suppression is the dose limiting toxicity. Other toxic effects include peripheral neuropathies, mucositis and hypersensitivity reactions.

❒❒ **What is asparaginase?**

An enzyme with anticancer activity. It was originally discovered in guinea pig serum.

❒❒ **What is the rationale behind using asparaginase in cancer therapy?**

A few neoplastic cells have low levels of asparagine synthetase activity and require L-asparagine for growth. Thus asparaginase hydrolyzes the amino acid making it unavailable for those cells.

❒❒ **What a type of cancer is asparaginase used to treat?**

It is used to induce remission in acute lymphocytic leukemia.

❑❑ What is the drawback of using asparaginase in cancer therapy?

Resistance rapidly develops to it.

❑❑ What is hydroxyurea?

A small molecular inhibitor of ribonucleotide reductase.

❑❑ What is the mechanism of action of hydroxyurea?

Inhibition of DNA synthesis.

❑❑ What are the therapeutic uses of hydroxyurea?

Chronic myelocytic leukemia (CML) and other myeloproliferative disorders.

❑❑ How are estrogens and its derivatives used in the treatment of cancer?

For the treatment of prostate cancer and advanced breast cancer in post-menopausal patients.

❑❑ What is the mechanism of action of tamoxifen?

It is an estrogen agonist and an antiestrogen. It is a competitive inhibitor of estradiol binding to the estrogen receptor. It decreases the autocrine stimulation of breast cancer growth.

❑❑ What are the therapeutic uses of tamoxifen?

It is used in breast cancer treatment and prevention, mostly in postmenopausal women.

❑❑ What are the toxic effects of tamoxifen?

Menopausal symptoms are most commonly seen (hot flashes etc.). Ocular toxicity, thromboembolic events, and endometrial cancer can also occur.

❑❑ What is flutamide?

A synthetic nonsteroidal antiandrogen.

❑❑ What is flutamide used for?

The treatment of prostate cancer.

❑❑ What are the adverse effects of flutamide?

GI effects, gynecomastia, and hepatotoxicity.

❒❒ Why are aromatase inhibitors useful in cancer?

They inhibit the final step in estrogen synthesis and thus are useful for the treatment of breast cancer.

❒❒ What are the toxic effects of the aromatase inhibitors?

GI disturbances are common. Other adverse effects include general weakness, nausea, headache and back pain.

❒❒ Name two selective aromatase inhibitors?

Anastrozole, letrozole and exemestane.

❒❒ How are these aromatase inhibitors used in breast cancer treatment?

They are used in postmenopausal women with disease progression after tamoxifen therapy.

IMMUNOPHARMACOLOGY

❒❒ What is meant by active immunotherapy?

You stimulate antitumor immunity specifically with vaccines or nonspecifically with other agents.

❒❒ What agents are used to stimulate passive immunity?

Biological response modifiers (BRMs).

❒❒ What diseases are treated with immunotherapy?

Cancer, multiple sclerosis, and chronic granulomatous disease.

❒❒ What type of cancer is interferon alpha used to treat?

Hematological malignancies and certain solid tumors.

❒❒ What is type of cancer is IL-2 used to treat?

Metastatic renal cell cancer and malignant melanoma and colorectal cancer.

❒❒ What are immunosuppressive drugs used for?

To prevent rejection during organ transplantation and to treat autoimmune diseases.

❒❒ What autoimmune diseases have produced the best results following immunosuppressive drug treatment?

Rheumatoid arthritis, Wegener's granulomatosis and the nephrotic syndrome in children.

❑❑ What are the undesirable effects of immunosuppressive therapy in general?

Nonselective depression of the host's immune system, severe drug toxicity (bone marrow suppression and GI effects etc.) and an increased incidence of malignancy.

❑❑ How do the steroids produce their immunosuppressive effect?

They act at multiple sites. They have an antiinflammatory action. They also disrupt intercellular communication among leukocytes through interference with production and function of lymphokines and they alter lymphocyte traffic and induce peripheral blood lymphopenia.

❑❑ How are the steroids used therapeutically as immunosuppressives?

They are used in combination to prevent and reverse allograft rejection and to treat various autoimmune diseases.

❑❑ What type of toxicity is associated with the use of steroids as immunosuppressives?

They are used in high doses and for prolonged times so the typical steroidal toxicities may occur e.g. osteoporosis, CNS effects.

❑❑ How is cyclophosphamide used as an immunosuppressive agent?

It is used to treat autoimmune diseases, as an alternate to drugs like imuran, in renal transplant patients especially in developing countries and in bone marrow transplants.

❑❑ What is azathioprine?

A prodrug of 6-mercaptopurine.

❑❑ Why is it more effective as an immunosuppressive than 6-MP?

Probably due to the slow release of 6-MP.

❑❑ How is azathioprine used as an immunosuppressive?

In combination regimens to prevent rejection in kidney transplant patients, and to treat several autoimmune disorders, most commonly rheumatoid arthritis.

❑❑ What toxicities are associated with the use of a zathioprine?

Bone marrow suppression and GI effects. Hepatotoxicity has also been reported with azathioprine.

❑❑ How does mycophenolic acid work?

It is a potent inhibitor of IMP dehydrogenase an enzyme critical for *de novo* purine synthesis. It also suppresses proliferation and inhibits the recruitment of leukocytes to inflammatory sites.

❑❑ What form is mycophenolic acid provided as?

It is provided as a prodrug ester, mycophenolate mofetil.

❑❑ What are the therapeutic uses of mycophenolic acid?

To prevent rejection in renal transplantation (it has replaced imuran in many areas).

❑❑ What toxicities are associated with the use of mycophenolic acid?

GI and bone marrow.

❑❑ What is the primary use of methotrexate as an immunosuppressive agent?

To treat rheumatoid arthritis.

❑❑ What are the advantages to the use of methotrexate in rheumatoid arthritis?

It is relatively well tolerated, has a low risk of carcinogenicity and has a long duration of response.

❑❑ What toxicities are of greatest concern when methotrexate is used to treat rheumatoid arthritis?

Pneumonitis and hepatotoxicity.

❑❑ Which monoclonal antibodies are now available to treat immunosuppressive disease?

Muromonab-CD3, basiliximab and daclizamab.

❑❑ What is muromonab-CD3?

A monoclonal antibody to the CD3 antigen of human T lymphocytes.

❑❑ How does muromonab-CD3 work?

It blocks the function and generation of cytotoxic T lymphocytes.

❑❑ What are the therapeutic uses of muromonab-CD3?

To prevent acute rejection of kidney, liver and heart transplants.

❑❑ What are the adverse effects of muromonab-CD3?

A cytokine release syndrome, anaphylactoid reactions, CNS effects and immunosuppression.

❑❑ What are basiliximab and daclizabab?

Mouse/human monoclonal antibodies that block the IL-2 receptor on T lymphocytes.

❑❑ How are these monoclonals used therapeutically?

To prevent acute renal transplant rejection.

❑❑ What is cyclosporine?

An immunosuppressive agent. It is a cyclic polypeptide containing some unique amino acids.

❑❑ What is the mechanism of action of cyclosporine?

It binds cyclophilin, an immunophilin, which then inhibits calcineurin a phosphatase. This results in inhibition of signal transduction pathways from the cytoplasm to the nucleus. It basically interrupts the cytokine activation cascade.

❑❑ How is cylcosporine administered?

It can be given orally or IV. A new oral microemulsion is now available which is the preferred oral formulation.

❑❑ What are the therapeutic uses of cyclosporine?

It is used mainly for the prevention and treatment of organ transplant rejection. Also it is used to treat several autoimmune diseases.

❑❑ What is the principal toxicity of cyclosporine?

Nephrotoxicity.

❑❑ What other toxic effects are associated with the use of cyclosporine?

Hypertension, neurotoxicity, hirsutism, hepatotoxicity, GI toxicity and gingival hyperplasia can all occur. Patients are also predisposed towards opportunistic infections and an increased incidence of lymphoma.

❑❑ What types of drug interactions is cylcosporine involved in?

Increases in nephrotoxicity occur when given with other nephrotoxic agents and drugs that affect the cytochrome p450 mixed function oxidase system can alter the metabolism of cyclosporine.

❑❑ What is tacrolimus?

It is a macrolide antibiotic immunosuppressive agent, which may be more potent than cyclosporine.

❑❑ What is the mechanism of action of tacrolimus?

It works very similarly to cyclosporine but it binds to a different immunophilin.

❏❏ How is tacrolimus used therapeutically?

It has similar uses to cyclosporine that is to prevent and treat organ graft rejection and in graft vs host disease in bone marrow transplantation.

❏❏ How does the toxicity of tacrolimus compare to cyclosporine?

Nephrotoxicity is the major problem. Hyperglycemia is more common as is neurotoxicity.

❏❏ What is sirolimus?

A macrolide immunosuppressive with a similar structure but different mechanism from tacrolimus.

❏❏ How does sirolimus work?

It binds to a cytosolic immunophilin and interferes with calcium independent pathways. It also blocks cytokine signal transduction pathways.

❏❏ How is sirolimus used therapeutically?

It is used for the prophylaxis of organ rejection in patients receiving renal transplants.

❏❏ What is the major toxicity of sirolimus?

Hyperlipidemia, hypertension and rash.

TOXICOLOGY

❑❑ What is toxicology?

It is the scientific discipline concerned with the deleterious effects of physical and chemical agents in living systems. It includes a description of toxic effects, mechanisms by which chemicals produce their effects, the environmental safety of chemicals and the legal and regulatory aspects of chemical safety.

❑❑ What is the LD50?

The dose lethal to 50% of the population. It is analogous to the ED50.

❑❑ What is meant by NOAEL and NOEL?

No observed effect level or no observed adverse effect level.

❑❑ What is the difference between acute toxicity, subacute toxicity and chronic toxicity?

Acute toxicity usually occurs after a single exposure to a large dose of chemical. It usually occurs within seconds to hours of the administration. Subacute toxicity occurs within days to months and chronic toxicity occurs within months to years.

❑❑ What types of toxicity testing are required for drugs and chemicals?

Acute toxicity, ninety day toxicity test, chronic or long-term toxicity and certain selected tests such as reproductive toxicity and mutagenesis.

❑❑ What are the problems associated with various toxicity testing procedures?

The extrapolation to humans and the dosage to be used in chronic testing.

❑❑ What is the general treatment of poisoned patients?

Maintain vital signs, minimize absorption, enhance elimination and use a specific antidote.

❑❑ What is the mechanism of carbon monoxide (CO) poisoning?

It binds reversibly to hemoglobin (specifically to the ferrous ion). The affinity of CO for hemoglobin is 240 times that for oxygen.

❑❑ What are the signs of CO intoxication?

Psychomotor impairment, headache and tightness in the temporal area, confusion and loss of visual acuity, deep coma, convulsions, shock and respiratory failure.

❑❑ How is CO intoxication treated?

Removal of the individual from the exposure and administration of oxygen.

❑❑ Why is sulfur dioxide toxic?

It forms sulfurous acid, which is an irritant to the eyes, mucus membranes etc. Extreme exposure can lead to pulmonary edema.

❑❑ How do nitrogen oxides produce toxicity?

They are lung irritants capable of producing pulmonary edema.

❑❑ How do you treat exposure from sulfur and nitrogen oxides?

There is no specific treatment but measures should be taken to reduce the risk of exposure.

❑❑ What is the toxicity of ozone thought to be due to?

It is an irritant to the mucus membranes and lungs. The toxicity is thought to result from free radical formation.

❑❑ How do you treat ozone toxicity?

There is no specific treatment for acute ozone toxicity. Management depends on therapeutic measures for deep lung irritation and noncardiogenic pulmonary edema.

❑❑ What is the mechanism of cyanide poisoning?

Cyanide poisoning results from complexing of cytochrome iron by the CN^- ion. Cytochrome oxidase is one of the targets.

❑❑ How is cyanide toxicity treated?

Methemoglobin iron has a high affinity for CN^- thus it is treated by converting ferrous iron of hemoglobin to ferric iron (methemoglobin). The methemoglobin binds cyanide ion to protect cytochromes and reverse the cytochrome cyanide binding.

❑❑ In general how do metals cause toxicity?

They form complexes with a number of natural functional groups like hydroxyl, carboxy, sulfhydryl, phosphate and amino groups. This binding leads to metal accumulation and redistribution. There may be non-specific enzyme inhibition and disruption of membrane function.

❑❑ What are the toxic forms of mercury?

The greatest danger is from organic mercury, although elemental mercury and inorganic salts all can produce toxicity.

❑❑ **In what organs is mercury toxic?**

Mercuric ion attacks the kidney primarily, producing acute tubular necrosis. Organic mercury compounds attack the CNS primarily and produce severe irreversible CNS damage.

❑❑ **Where and why is lead toxic?**

Lead can produce peripheral nerve damage, lead encephalopathy, kidney disease and anemia due to blockade of heme synthesis.

❑❑ **Where is cadmium toxicity produced?**

It can produce renal damage, emphysema like syndrome and osteomalacia in women.

❑❑ **Which form of arsenic is toxic?**

Trivalent arsenic compounds.

❑❑ **In what organs is arsenic toxicity seen?**

Acute poisoning to the GI, cardiopulmonary and CNS effects. Chronic poisoning produces peripheral neuropathy and hyperkeratosis and pigment changes in the skin.

❑❑ **What is the mechanism of action of arsenic?**

Pentavalent arsenic interferes with oxidative phosphorylation. Trivalent arsenicals are primarily sulfhydryl reagents.

❑❑ **How is acute arsenic toxicity treated?**

Gastric lavage, administration of dimercaprol or penicillamine and hemodialysis if there is renal failure.

❑❑ **How are the toxic effects of metals counteracted?**

With the use of chelating agents.

❑❑ **What are dimercaprol or BAL used for?**

Treatment of mercury and gold poisoning.

❑❑ **What is penicillamine used for?**

Treatment of copper, mercury and lead poisoning.

❑❑ **How is penicillamine given?**

Orally, it is the only commercially available oral chelating agent for adults.

❑❑ **What is deferoxamine used for?**

Treatment of iron toxicity.

❑❑ **How is deferoxamine administered?**

Parenterally.

❑❑ **What is calcium disodium edetate (EDTA) used for?**

Treatment of lead poisoning.

❑❑ **What is the major adverse effect associated with EDTA?**

Nephrotoxicity.

❑❑ **Why is methanol toxic?**

It produces systemic acidosis and blindness caused by the formaldehyde and formic acid.

❑❑ **How is methanol toxicity treated?**

Correction of the acidosis is the keystone to therapy. Ethanol can counter the metabolic acidosis.

❑❑ **What is the source of many hydrocarbon poisons?**

Industrial and cleaning solvents.

❑❑ **What are the toxic effects of kerosene?**

It produces CNS depression. It can also produce severe lung damage when it gets into the lung including chemical pneumonitis and pulmonary edema.

❑❑ **How is kerosene poisoning treated?**

Remove the patient from the source of exposure and provide supportive therapies.

❑❑ **What are the toxic effects of benzene?**

The acute toxic effect is CNS depression. Chronic exposure can lead to bone marrow depression. It is also carcinogenic in humans causing leukemia.

❑❑ **How is benzene toxicity treated?**

There is no specific treatment for acute benzene toxicity.

❑❑ What is the toxic form of carbon tetrachloride and chloroform?

They are toxic after metabolism. Carbon tetrachloride is converted to a trichloromethyl free radical leading to liver and renal damage. Chloroform is converted to phosgene leading to renal damage.

ENDOCRINE PHARMACOLOGY

❑❑ **What is ACTH and from where is it obtained?**

ACTH is adrenocorticotrophin or adrenocorticotrophic hormone. It is isolated from porcine pituitary or prepared as a newer synthetic hormone referred to as cosyntropin.

❑❑ **How is ACTH used?**

It is used for the diagnosis of hypothalamic pituitary axis dysfunction

❑❑ **What are somatrem and somatropin?**

They are recombinant human growth hormones. They are used for growth hormone deficiency as well as for Turner's syndrome, delayed growth, normal short stature and wound healing in large cutaneous burns.

❑❑ **What is protirelin and how is it used?**

It is a synthetic thyrotropin releasing hormone. It is used in the diagnosis of thyroid disease.

❑❑ **What is sermorelin and how is it used?**

It is synthetic growth hormone releasing hormone. It is used similarly to growth hormone, but it is ineffective in patients with a pituitary defect.

❑❑ **What is octreotide?**

A synthetic 8-aminoacid cyclic peptide analog of somatotropin.

❑❑ **What are the uses for octreotide?**

It is used for the treatment of hormone-secreting tumors. It is also effective for acromegaly due to growth hormone -secreting adenoma and adenomas secreting thyroid stimulating hormone or glucagon and certain GI-secretion disorders.

❑❑ **What is bromocriptine and how is it used?**

It is a dopamine agonist analog used to treat hyperprolactinemia, prolactinomas (prolactin secreting adenomas), and for suppression of lactation. It also inhibits growth hormone and is useful in acromegaly.

❑❑ **What is vasopressin?**

A 9 amino acid peptide hormone released in response to increased plasma osmolarity or decreased blood pressure.

❒❒ What is the mechanism of action of vasopressin?

It acts on V-1 receptors of vascular smooth muscle to cause vasoconstriction and on V-2 receptors of kidney to promote water reabsorption in collecting tubules. V-2 receptors also increase blood clotting by increasing release of Von Willebrands's factor and Factor VIII.

❒❒ What is vasopressin used for?

Vasopressin deficiency results in diabetes insipidus; vasopressin or its analogs are used as replacement therapy.

❒❒ What synthetic versions of vasopressin are available?

Arginine vasopressin is a synthetic version of the natural hormone. It is the agent of choice for V-1 receptor related applications. Lypressin is a more stable analog with a longer half-life and desmopressin is a long acting synthetic analog with a high ratio of antidiuretic to pressor activity.

❒❒ What is desmopressin used for and how is it given?

It can be inhaled, injected IV or SC and given orally. It is used for most cases of diabetes insipidus. Other uses include nocturnal enuresis, hemophilia, and von Willebrands disease.

❒❒ What are the side effects of vasopressin and its analogs?

Increased blood pressure, GI and uterine contractions, cramps, headache, and nausea.

❒❒ What is oxytocin and how does it differ from vasopressin?

It is a 9 amino acid cyclic peptide, differing from vasopressin by two amino acids.

❒❒ How is oxytocin administered?

IV, IM, or by nasal spray.

❒❒ What is oxytocin used for?

It is used to induce labor and augment dysfunctional labor. It can also be used for control of postpartum uterine hemorrhage. It can also be used diagnostically to indicate intrauterine growth retardation.

❒❒ How is the secretion of the thyroid hormones regulated?

Thyrotropin releasing hormone (TRH) from the hypothalamus controls release of thyrotropin from the anterior pituitary, which regulates synthesis and release of thyroid hormones. T3(triiodothyronine) and T4 (thyroxine) feedback on the hypothalamus and pituitary to inhibit release, therefore maintaining tight control of hormone levels. Iodine availability also regulates thyroid hormone production with high iodine inhibiting synthesis.

❑❑ How and where are T3 and T4 synthesized?

They are synthesized in the thyroid gland, iodide is taken up and oxidized by peroxidase, attached to protein thyroglobulin as mono- and di-iodotyrosine and conjugated to form T3 and T4. They are stored in colloid and through endocytosis and proteolysis of thyroglobulin T3 and T4 are released.

❑❑ How do T3 and T4 differ?

T4 is more protein bound than T3 while T3 is more rapidly metabolized and is more potent than T4.

❑❑ What type of receptor is there for the thyroid hormones T3 and T4?

Both act on the same receptor to produce the same effect. The receptor is a nuclear transcription regulator similar to the steroid hormone receptors and regulates specific thyroid hormone response elements.

❑❑ What are the main uses of thyroid hormones?

They are mainly used as replacement therapy in hypothyroidism.

❑❑ Which is the primary drug used for hypothyroidism?

Thyroxine (T4).

❑❑ Why is T3 rarely used?

It has a very rapid onset and consequently marked physiological effects. It also has a short half-life.

❑❑ What are the side effects of the thyroid hormones?

Symptoms of hyperthyroidism such as increased metabolism, catecholamine potentiation, diarrhea, weakness, tiredness, decreased concentration, amenorrhea and exophthalmos.

❑❑ How is hyperthyroidism treated?

With the use of anti-thyroid drugs, therapeutic radioiodine or partial thyroidectomy.

❑❑ What are the uses for the thioamides?

They are first line therapy for hyperthyroidism.

❑❑ What are the names of the two thioamides used in therapy?

Methimazole and propylthiouracil.

❑❑ **Why is methimazole the drug of choice among the thioamides?**

It has a longer half-life than propylthiouracil and thus can be used once a day.

❑❑ **What is the mechanism of action of the thioamides?**

They act through multiple mechanisms. The major action is to prevent hormone synthesis by inhibiting the thyroid peroxidase-catalyzed reactions to block iodine organification. In addition they block coupling of the iodotyrosines.

❑❑ **What are the major adverse effects of the thioamides?**

The most common adverse effect is a maculopapular pruritic rash. The most dangerous complication is agranulocytosis.

❑❑ **How are the iodides used?**

They are only used therapeutically in the immediate pre-op period in preparation for subtotal thryoidectomy and in the treatment of thyroid storm.

❑❑ **What adverse effects are associated with the use of iodides?**

Adverse reactions are uncommon and in most cases reversible upon discontinuance. They include sore throat, burning mouth, metallic taste, bleeding disorders, rash and diarrhea.

❑❑ **What is the use for radioactive iodine?**

Small doses are used in tracer studies of I^{131} uptake for diagnosis of hyperthyroidism, anatomy and function of thyroid tissue and localization of metastatic thyroid cancer. Larger doses are used for destruction of tissue.

❑❑ **What is the treatment of choice for hyperthyroidism?**

It depends on the age, presence of pregnancy, surgical risk of the patient and the size, severity, duration and pathophysiology of the hyperthyroidism.

❑❑ **What is thyroid storm?**

A massive release of thyroid hormone.

❑❑ **How is thyroid storm treated?**

Propylthiouracil is given to prevent conversion of T4 to T3; Iodide is used to decrease the release of thyroid hormones; and glucocorticoids are used to prevent shock. The conversion of T3 to T4 has to be slowed and symptomatic relief (e.g. propranolol or diltiazem to decrease sympathetic effects.) is also used.

❑❑ **What is diabetes mellitus?**

A syndrome charecterized by various metabolic disturbances and inappropriate hyperglycemia.

❑❑ What is the difference between Type 1 diabetes and Type 2 diabetes?

Type 1 or insulin dependent diabetes (IDDM) is a severe form associated with ketosis in the untreated state. It is most common in juveniles, but occasionally occurs in adults. In IDDM circulating insulin is nearly absent, plasma glucagon is raised, and the pancreatic B cell fail to respond to all insulinogenic stimuli. The basic defect is thought to be an autoimmune destruction of insulin secreting B cells.

Type 2 or non-insulin dependent diabetes (NIDDM) is a milder form of diabetes that occurs chiefly in adults. Circulating insulin is adequate to prevent ketoacidosis but is often either below normal or inadequate because of a decreased tissue response. Obesity is a common risk factor. There are various genetic defects in insulin secretion and response.

❑❑ What is the treatment for insulin dependent diabetes (Type 1)?

The treatment includes parenteral insulin as well as dietary control and exercise.

❑❑ What is the treatment for non-insulin dependent diabetes (Type 2)?

Oral hypoglycemic agents, dietary modification, weight reduction and parenteral insulin in those situations where there is no response to the other treatments.

❑❑ What is insulin?

A 51 amino acid peptide produced in the beta cells of the pancreas.

❑❑ What are the major actions of insulin?

It produces increased glucose uptake by fat and muscle, increased glucose storage as glycogen, decreased glycogenolysis, increased glycolysis, decreased gluconeogenesis, increased amino acid uptake and protein synthesis, decreased protein degradation, increased lipid synthesis and growth factor like effects.

❑❑ What is the mechanism of insulin's effects?

It acts on a cell surface receptor linked to multiple second messengers? There is tyrosine kinase activation, changes in cyclic AMP, phosphoinositide hydrolysis, phosphorylation of metabolic enzymes, glucose transporter translocation and nuclear effects.

❑❑ What is glucagon?

Glucagon is a 29 amino acid peptide synthesized in the A cells of the pancreatic islets of Langerhans.

❑❑ What does glucagon do?

It is released from the pancreas in response to hypoglycemia. It increases glucose by the opposite effects of insulin. Its immediate effect is to raise blood glucose at the expense of stored hepatic glycogen. It also causes release of insulin from normal pancreatic B cells.

❑❑ What is the mechanism of action of glucagon?

It binds to specific receptors on liver cells and this leads to a G protein linked increase in adenylyl cyclase activity and the production of cAMP which facilitates catabolism of stored glycogen and increases gluconeogenesis and ketogenesis.

❑❑ What are the three main classes of insulin?

Short acting (insulin lispro and regular), intermediate acting (isophane insulin suspension and insulin zinc suspension-lente) and long acting (insulin zinc suspension-ultralente).

❑❑ How do the different insulin preparations compare as far as efficacy?

All the preparations have equal efficacy but important pharmacokinetic differences.

❑❑ What are the differences between lente, semilente and ultralente insulins.

Onset and duration of action. Ultralente has the longest duration.

❑❑ What is the advantage of ultralente insulin?

It provides better control between meals and better overnight control.

❑❑ What is the advantage of the short acting regular insulin?

It provides more immediate effects for premeal use.

❑❑ What are the drawbacks of regular insulin?

It has a short duration and thus requires more frequent injections..

❑❑ How does insulin lispro differ from the other insulins?

It is a recombinant preparation with LysPro rather than normal ProLys. It aggregates less so it is absorbed faster. Its kinetics most closely resembles the physiological situation. It can be injected immediately before meals so the timing of meals is less critical.

❑❑ What are the adverse effects of insulin?

They are mainly hypoglycemia, but less commonly immunologic reactions occur. Also atrophy of subcutaneous fat at the site of insulin injection (lipoatrophy) and lipohypertrophy.

❑❑ What kinds of drugs will interact with insulin?

A large number of drugs can cause hypoglycemia or hyperglycemia or may alter a diabetic patient response to therapy. Among the most common drugs producing hypoglycemia are ethanol, beta-adrenergic receptor antagonists and salicylates. There are also many drugs which can cause hyperglycemia in normal people or impair metabolic control in diabetics, many of which have direct effects on peripheral tissues that counter the actions of insulin (e.g. epinephrine, glucocorticoids and oral contraceptives). Some drugs inhibit insulin secretion directly or indirectly (e.g. phenytoin, calcium channel blockers and diuretics).

❑❑ What effects do propranolol and other beta-blockers have on insulin use?

They mask the symptoms of hypoglycemia.

❑❑ Should insulin be used in pregnancy?

It is preferred in pregnancy to the oral agents.

❑❑ What types of diabetes are the oral hypoglycemic agents used in?

They are used alone or with insulin or other oral agents in type II diabetes only.

❑❑ Name two first and two second generation sulfonylureas?

Chlorpropamide and tolbutamide are first generation sulfonylureas while glyburide, glipizide and glimepiride are second generation compounds.

❑❑ What is the advantage of the second-generation sulfonylureas over the first generation compounds?

They are safer and more potent.

❑❑ What is the mechanism of action of the sulfonylureas?

They increase insulin secretion by the beta cells. They are ATP sensitive K^+ channel blockers. They lead to depolarization, Ca^{2+} influx and increased insulin secretion and they have secondary effects decreasing glucagon and increasing tissue sensitivity to insulin.

❑❑ Compare the use of glyburide with glipizide.

Glipizide has the shortest half-life and may be better for post-prandial hyperglycemia and daytime use and the longer acting glyburide may be better for fasting effects and overnight use.

❑❑ Can the sulfonylureas be used in kidney or liver disease?

They are dangerous to be used in these situations.

❑❑ What are the adverse effects of the sulfonylureas?

Hypoglycemia due to an overdose, occasional GI distress, pruritis, nausea, agranulocytosis and aplastic anemia (rare).

❑❑ Do the second-generation sulfonylureas have an increased or decreased incidence of adverse effects compared to the first generation compounds?

The second generation compounds produce adverse effects slightly less frequently.

❑❑ What drug-drug interactions are involved with the sulfonylureas?

Several compounds augment the hypoglycemic effect of these drugs. They include NSAIDS, alcohol and some antibacterials. Diuretics and corticosteroids decrease the action of these drugs.

❑❑ What is repaglinide?

A relatively new oral antidiabetic agent related to the sulfonylureas.

❑❑ How does repaglinide work?

It is structurally different from the sulfonylureas but also binds ATP sensitive potassium channels and increases insulin secretion.

❑❑ What is the advantage if any of repaglinide over the sulfonylureas?

It maybe safer than the sulfonylureas in kidney disease and may be less likely to cause hypoglycemia.

❑❑ What is metformin?

A biguanide compound used to treat hyperglycemia.

❑❑ What is the mechanism of action of metformin?

It decreases glucose production (gluconeogenesis) but increases its uptake. It also increases the effectiveness of insulin. It also may reduce plasma glucagon levels.

❑❑ What is the major advantage of metformin over other oral hypoglycemic agents?

It does not cause hypoglycemia.

❑❑ What are the adverse effects of metformin?

The most frequent toxic effects are gastrointestinal (anorexia, nausea, vomiting, abdominal discomfort). Lactic acidosis can also occur.

❑❑ What is acarbose?

It is a complex microbial oligosaccharide that is poorly absorbed and thus remains in the gut.

❑❑ What is the mechanism of action of acarbose?

It inhibits α-glucosidase an intestinal disaccharidase. Absorption of most carbohydrates including starches, dextrins, maltose and sucrose, but not lactose is delayed.

❑❑ What adverse effects are associated with the use of acarbose?

The principal adverse effect is flatulence but diarrhea also occurs.

❑❑ What is troglitazone?

The first member of a new class of oral antidiabetics, referred to as thiazolidinedione derivatives.

❑❑ What is the mechanism of action of troglitazone?

It decreases gluconeogenesis, glucose output and triglyceride synthesis in the liver. It increases glucose uptake and utilization in muscle; increases glucose uptake and decreases fatty acid production in adipocytes. It acts by binding to nuclear peroxisome proliferator activated receptor This enhances transcription of insulin-responsive genes, regulates adipocyte differentiation and lipid and glucose metabolism.

❑❑ What advantages do rosiglitazone and pioglitazone have over troglitazone?

They are newer members of the thiazolidinediones and may lack toxicity to the liver.

❑❑ Which is the oral calcium preparation containing the highest percent of calcium?

Calcium carbonate.

❑❑ What is the calcium preparation least irritating to veins and thus the drug of choice for IV therapy?

Calcium gluconate.

❑❑ What is the only parenteral calcium preparation not irritating upon IM injection?

Calcium gluceptate.

❑❑ Describe the actions of parathyroid hormone?

It increases blood calcium, by increasing reabsorption of calcium from the kidney and increases absorption of both calcium and phosphate from the GI tract.

❑❑ Is parathyroid hormone used therapeutically?

There are no current therapeutic uses, but it is used diagnostically in hypothyroidism.

❑❑ What is needed to insure absorption of calcium preparations?

Adequate vitamin D.

❑❑ What are the actions of vitamin D?

It increases blood calcium and phosphate by enhancing resorption of calcium and phosphate from bone, increases their absorption from the GI tract and may increase reabsorption of calcium and phosphate from the kidney.

❑❑ What is the form of vitamin D in foods?

Cholecalciferol and ergocalciferol.

❑❑ What is the effect of vitamin D in excess?

It can cause hypercalcemia and hypercalcuria.

❑❑ What is calcitriol?

The active vitamin D hormone. Clinically it is most important as it works in all patients.

❑❑ How is dihydrotachysterol used?

It is a reduced form of vitamin D_2 and is useful in renal failure, as it does not require renal hydroxylation.

❑❑ How is calcifediol used?

It does not require liver hydroxylation, so it is useful in liver disease.

❑❑ What is calcipotriene?

A vitamin D_3 analog available in a skin ointment for the treatment of psoriasis.

❑❑ What is calcitonin?

A 32 aminoacid polypeptide hormone produced in the parafollicular C cells of the thyroid gland. It is secreted in response to hypercalcemia and acts to decrease calcium levels.

❑❑ What are the effects of calcitonin?

It decreases blood calcium and phosphate. It acts on the bone to inhibit osteoclasts and on the kidney to increase excretion of calcium and phosphate.

❑❑ In what form is calcitonin available clinically?

It is available as synthetic salmon calcitonin and synthetic human calcitonin.

❑❑ What is the difference between synthetic salmon calcitonin and synthetic human calcitonin?

The salmon calcitonin is more potent and longer acting than the human preparation due to slower clearance. It is thus better for acute hypercalcemia. The human calcitonin is better for long-term antigenicity studies.

❑❑ **What are the biphosphonates?**

They are structural analogs of pyrophosphate. They inhibit osteoclasts and decrease bone turnover.

❑❑ **What are the therapeutic uses of the biphosphonates?**

They have similar uses to calcitonin e.g. Paget's disease, hypercalcemia, and osteoporosis.

❑❑ **What are the adverse effects of the biphosphonates?**

They cause gastric irritation with resulting occasional abdominal pain, nausea, diarrhea, and vomiting.

❑❑ **What is the difference between etidronate, pamidronate, alendronate and tiludronate?**

Etidronate was the first of the bisphosphonates and inhibits bone degradation but also inhibits mineralization. Pamidronate has less effect on bone mineralization and the last two have almost no effect on mineralization.

❑❑ **What is gallium nitrate used for?**

This agent inhibits bone resorption and is used for hypercalcemia, Paget's disease and osteoporosis.

❑❑ **What toxicity is associated with use of gallium nitrate?**

There is a potential for nephrotoxicity.

❑❑ **What is the mechanism of action of mithramycin?**

Mithramycin decreases plasma calcium. It has osteoclast toxicity that leads to decreased bone resorption.

❑❑ **What type of toxicity is associated with the use of mithramycin?**

The most dangerous toxic effect is sudden thrombocytopenia followed by hemorrhage. Hepatic and renal toxicity can also occur. Hypocalcemia, nausea and vomiting may limit therapy. It is a very toxic agent and can cause bone marrow depression.

❑❑ **What is mithramycin used for clinically?**

It is a second choice drug for treatment of hypercalcemia.

❑❑ **How does fluoride work?**

It stimulates osteoblasts and increases bone formation but it can also increase bone fragility at higher doses.

❒❒ What adverse effects does fluoride have if any?

It can result in inhibition of respiratory and glycolytic enzymes.

❒❒ What are the two major groups of corticosteroids?

Mineralocorticoids and glucocorticoids.

❒❒ What is the major site of production of the corticosteroids?

In the adrenal cortex.

❒❒ What is the primary endogenous glucocorticoid?

Cortisol.

❒❒ What are the primary metabolic effects of the glucocorticoids?

They effect several metabolic pathways. For example they produce an increase in blood glucose, an increase in protein catabolism in all tissues and a mobilization of fat from adipose tissue along with a redistribution of fat from the periphery to the trunk.

❒❒ What are the primary effects of the mineralocorticoids?

They control body fluid and electrolyte levels. There is an increase in sodium reabsorption; increased H^+ and K^+ excretion and activation of the renin-angiotensin system.

❒❒ Describe the anti-inflammatory and immunosuppressive effects of the mineralocorticoids?

They inhibit formation of arachidonic acid metabolites, there is a reduction of fever and pain. There is inhibition of prostaglandin and leukotriene release from macrophages, monocytes, endothelial cells, and fibroblasts. There is also enhancement of vasoconstriction and a decrease in vascular permeability. There is an increase in peripheral neutrophils and a decrease in peripheral T and B lymphocytes and an inhibition of phagocytosis. There also is decreased production of several cytokines and other inflammatory mediators.

❒❒ What is the mechanism of action of the steroid hormones?

They enter the cell and bind to specific cytosolic receptors. The hormone complex then enters the nucleus and binds to specific sites on DNA to enhance transcription of specific genes, which leads to synthesis of specific proteins.

❒❒ What are the principle glucocorticoids available?

Hydrocortisone, cortisone, prednisolone, prednisone, triamcinolone and dexamethasone.

❒❒ Compare hydrocortisone to prednisone and dexamethasone with regard to potency, relative anti-inflammatory action, relative sodium retaining potency, plasma half-life and biological half-life?

Hydrocortisone is the least potent of the three, while dexamethasone is the most potent. The same is true for anti-inflammatory potency and sodium retaining potency. Dexamethasone has the longest plasma half-life and biological half-life and hydrocortisone the least.

❒❒ Why is the biological half-life of the glucocorticoids longer than the plasma half-life?

It is due to sequestration in tissues and the slow turnover of proteins.

❒❒ How are the glucocorticoids administered?

Numerous ways, including oral, parenteral and various preparations for local administration.

❒❒ What are some of the anti-inflammatory and immunosuppressive uses of the glucocorticoids?

Arthritis, bursitis, collagen vascular diseases, skin diseases, asthma, renal diseases, ulcerative colitis, inflammatory bowel disease, eye disease, prevention of organ or graft rejection etc.

❒❒ What are the adverse effects of the glucocorticoids?

A number of adverse effects are produced by long term use of these agents. They include mineralocorticoid effects such as edema, hypernatremia, hypokalemia, alkalosis, and hypertension.

They also produce glucocorticoid effects like muscle wasting, weakness, skin thinning, osteoporosis, inhibition of growth; diabetes or insulin resistance, weight gain, fat redistribution; stimulation of peptic ulcer, CNS disturbances such as psychosis or euphoria; cataracts; glaucoma; poor wound healing and an increased risk of infection.

❒❒ Under what conditions must glucocorticoids be used with great caution?

As a result of their effects they must be used with great caution in heart disease, hypertension, diabetes, peptic ulcer, infections, osteoporosis, glaucoma, psychoses.

❒❒ What are the best ways to use the glucocorticoids as antiinflammatory agents in order to avoid toxicity?

Use them over the short term with high doses, and use as a last resort. Also use the smallest effective dose, and give by localized administration, alternate day administration and cyclical administration. They should be withdrawn slowly when the regimen is complete.

❑❑ How are the glucocorticoids used as replacement therapy?

They are used in primary adrenal insufficiency (Addison's disease) in secondary insufficienty due to defective anterior pituitary or hypothalamic function or in acute situations due to abrupt withdrawal or with stress in adrenally compromised patients.

❑❑ Which glucocorticoid should be used as replacement therapy?

Hydrocortisone is useful since both glucocorticoid and mineralocorticoid effects may be needed. You may have to supplement it with fludrocortisone for additional mineralocorticoid effects if needed.

❑❑ What is meant by congenital adrenal hyperplasia?

This is a defect in the enzymes of cortisol synthesis with a compensatory increase in ACTH that leads to hyperplasia of the adrenal cortex and an increase in all precursos in the pathways not affected by the block.

❑❑ How is congenital adrenal hyperplasia treated?

Treat with a glucocorticoid to replace the missing cortisol to reverse ACTH overproduction and suppress excess androgen and/or mineralocorticoid secretion.

❑❑ What are the two naturally occurring mineralocorticoids?

Aldosterone and deoxycorticosterone.

❑❑ What is the normal physiological function of aldosterone?

It acts on the renal tubule cells to increase reabsorption of sodium, bicarbonate and water in exchange for potassium excretion.

❑❑ Which mineralocorticoid is most commonly used in therapy?

Fludrocortisone.

❑❑ What is fludrocortisone used for?

Replacement therapy after adrenalectomy or for primary and secondary adrenocortical insufficiency.

❑❑ What adverse effects are seen with fludrocortisone therapy?

Hypokalemia and congestive heart failure.

❑❑ What is spironolactone?

An orally effective aldosterone antagonist that also has anti-androgenic effects.

❑❑ How is spironolactone used clinically?

For the treatment of aldosterone secreting tumors and in the treatment of hirsutism.

❏❏ What is metyrapone and what is it used for?

It is an inhibitor of the 11-hydroxylase enzyme and reduces cortisol production. It is used to diagnose adrenal insufficiency and Cushings syndrome and in the treatment of adrenal carcinoma or ectopic ACTH production.

❏❏ What is aminoglutethimide and what is it used for?

It inhibits the first step in corticosteroid biosynthesis and therefore inhibits synthesis of all adrenal steroids. It is used in patients who have Cushing's syndrome and in hormone-dependent cancers.

❏❏ How does ketoconazole effect steroid synthesis and how is it used?

It blocks the heme site in cytochrome P-450 enzymes (e.g.11-hydroxylase) required for glucocorticoid synthesis. It has some use in Cushing's syndrome due to malignancy and other causes.

❏❏ What is mifepristone and how is it used?

A new glucocorticoid and progesterone receptor antagonist. It has been used experimentally in the treatment of Cushing's syndrome and has been used as an abortifacient.

❏❏ What are the major categories of sex steroids?

Estrogens, progestins and androgens.

❏❏ What is the primary female sex hormone in humans?

Estradiol-17β.

❏❏ What is the primary hormone in humans that promotes gestation?

Progesterone.

❏❏ What is the primary male sex hormone in humans?

Testosterone.

❏❏ What are the precursors to estrogen synthesis?

Androstenedione and testosterone.

❏❏ Why are the native sex hormones inactive orally?

Due to poor absorption and/or rapid metabolism.

❑❑ **What are the active metabolites of estradiol?**

Estrone and estriol.

❑❑ **What is the active species of testosterone in many tissues?**

Dihydrotestosterone.

❑❑ **How are the production of these sex hormones controlled?**

Control is by gonadotropins from the anterior pituitary, which in turn is under control of gonadotropin-releasing hormones from the hypothalamus. There is a complex feedback regulation.

❑❑ **What is the mechanism of action of the steroid hormones?**

Free steroid crosses the cell membrane and binds to intracellular nuclear receptors. The receptor-hormone complex induces or represses transcription of specific genes by binding to steroid response elements on DNA. There are separate estrogen, progesterone and androgen receptors and response elements, which results in specificity.

❑❑ **What are the most important physiological effects of the estrogens?**

Growth and development of internal and external genitalia, development of breasts, female figure and skin texture., growth stimulation, and closure of the epiphyses of long bones. As far as metabolic effects there is decreased bone resorption, altered lipid metabolism (decreased total and LDL cholesterol, increased HDL cholesterol and triglycerides) and altered protein synthesis (increased levels of binding globulins for many steroids, increased synthesis of blood clotting factors and angiotensinogen).

❑❑ **What estrogens are available commercially?**

Estradiol, conjugated estrogens, ethinyl estradiol and mestranol.

❑❑ **How is estradiol administered?**

Estradiol itself is ineffective orally due to first pass metabolism by the liver. There is a micronized oral preparation available as well as topical preparations and a slow-release depot form for IM injection.

❑❑ **What are the conjugated estrogens?**

Ester conjugates and salts of estrone and estriol isolated from pregnant mare urine.

❑❑ **What is the major use of the conjugated estrogens?**

Hormone replacement therapy.

❑❑ **What is ethinyl estradiol?**

A synthetic estrogen preparation with an attached ethinyl group which greatly slows its metabolism, increasing the potency and oral effectiveness. Mestranol is a prodrug of ethinyl estradiol.

❑❑ What is the common use for mestranol and ethinyl estradiol?

As oral contraceptives.

❑❑ Name two nonsteroidal estrogens?

Diethylstilbestrol and dienestrol.

❑❑ What are the clinical uses of the estrogens?

As oral contraceptives (combined with progestins). For the treatment of hypogonadism, hypopituitarism (replacement therapy). For post-menopausal hormone replacement therapy (with progestins) and also for similar symptoms following oophorectomy.

❑❑ What is raloxifene?

A tissue specific estrogen with beneficial effects on bone and heart disease without unwanted effects on reproductive tissue.

❑❑ What are the toxic effects of estrogen use?

Nausea and edema are most common. Other effects include breast tenderness, hyperpigmentation, migraine, hypertension, cholestasis, and gall bladder disease. At high doses there may be thrombophlebitis and thromboembolic complications. Endometrial hyperplasia and an increased risk of endometrial cancer (risk is reduced by including progestins). In men there may be gynecomastia and feminization.

❑❑ What is tamoxifen?

A nonsteroidal estrogen with mixed agonist/antagonist properties.

❑❑ What is tamoxifen used for

To treat and prevent breast cancer especially in postmenopausal women.

❑❑ What is clomiphene?

A non-steroidal weak agonist used as an antagonist. It blocks feedback receptors and increases gonadotropin release.

❑❑ What is clomiphene used for?

To stimulate ovulation in patients who want to become pregnant.

❑❑ What is danazol?

A weak androgen and progestin. It inhibits gonadotropin secretion and steroid synthesis.

❑❑ How is danazol used?

It is used mainly for its anti-estrogenic effects. It is given orally and is used in the treatment of endometriosis and fibrocystic breast disease.

❑❑ What are the gonadotropin releasing hormone (GnRH) agonist analogs?

They are modified synthetic peptides with long durations of action. They are injected daily or given as depot preparations to inhibit gonadotropin release.

❑❑ How are the GnRH agonist analogs used clinically?

They are used for their antiestrogenic effects in breast cancer, endometriosis, uterine fibroids and polycystic ovary syndrome. They are also used as anti-androgens in prostate cancer, hirsutism, and for precocious puberty in both sexes.

❑❑ Name one of the GnRH analogs?

Leuprolide.

❑❑ What are the two types of progestins used clinically?

Those structurally related to progesterone and those structurally related to testosterone.

❑❑ Name three progesterones that are closely related to progesterone?

Medroxyprogesterone acetate, hydroxyprogtesterone acetate and megestrol acetate.

❑❑ Name three progesterones that are related to testosterone?

Norethindrone, norgestrel, ethynodiol.

❑❑ What are the therapeutic uses of the progestins?

They are used as contraceptives (alone or with estrogens) for postmenopausal hormone replacement therapy (with estrogens) for dysfunctional uterine bleeding due to endometrial hyperplasia for endometriosis and accompanying dysmenorrea and for diagnostic evaluation of estrogen secretion and endometrial responsiveness.

❑❑ What are the adverse effects of the progestins?

With the androgenic progestins there may be acne, weight gain, masculinization, decreased HDL, increased LDL. All progestins can produce menstrual changes, nausea, bloating and teratogenesis.

❑❑ Name an antiprogestin drug?

Mifepristone.

❑❑ What two types of oral contraceptives are available in the U.S.?

Combination oral contraceptives that contain both an estrogen and a progestin, and progestin-only contraceptives (mini-pills).

❑❑ Which type of oral contraceptive is most effective?

When used as directed all oral contraceptives marketed in the U.S. are similarly effective.

❑❑ What types of contraceptives are most commonly used today?

The combination contraceptives with ethinyl estradiol or mestranol plus a 19-nor progestin are commonly used.

❑❑ What do the terms monophasic and multiphasic mean regarding the oral contraceptives?

Monophasic oral contraceptives refer to those containing fixed doses of estrogen and progestin in each pill while multiphasic oral contraceptives have varying doses of one or both hormones during the cycle.

❑❑ How are the combination contraceptives given?

They are taken for 21 days and then a placebo or no pill is taken for 7 days during which menstruation occurs.

❑❑ How do the various oral contraceptive preparations differ from each other?

There are varying levels of the estrogen component. There are also differences in the amount and properties of the progestin component. Some preparations contain constant levels of both hormones while others contain variable levels. There is a trend towards lower levels of both estrogen and progestin to reduce side effects.

❑❑ What is the mechanism of action of the oral contraceptives?

They inhibit ovulation by disrupting the cyclical release of gonadotropins. There are changes in cervical mucus, the endometrium, motility and secretions of fallopian tubes that decrease the likelihood of fertilization. Endometrial changes also occur that decrease likelihood of successful implantation. The abrupt withdrawal of progestin support of the endometrium at day 21 promotes prompt and physiological bleeding.

❑❑ What are the adverse effects of the combination pills?

There are relatively minor effects like nausea, headache, fluid retention, breast tenderness and enlargement, menstrual changes, altered libido, acne, weight gain, and hirsutism. Cardiovascular changes may also occur. The early high-dose pills caused increases in blood pressure, changes in serum lipid, increases in clotting factors, endothelial cell proliferation and decreases in blood flow. These changes led to an increased risk of thromboembolism, stoke and myocardial infarction. Although the estrogens alone increase the risk of endometrial cancer the combination pills may actually decrease the incidence of endometrial cancer and ovarian cancer. There may also be some metabolic changes such as mild glucose intolerance, altered hepatic lipid metabolism (progestins can cause unfavorable changes in LDL and HDL cholesterol), increased risk of liver and gall bladder disease although it is less with current pills. Teratogenesis is also possible and these pills should be discontinued if pregnancy is suspected.

❒❒ What are the beneficial effects of the oral contraceptives besides use in contraception?

A decrease in endometrial and ovarian cancer, a decrease in fibrocystic breast disease, ovarian cysts, endometriosis, pelvic inflammatory disease, iron deficiency anemia. There is also improved cycle regularity and decrease in premenstrual symptoms, menorrhagia and dysmenorrhea and increased spinal bone density.

❒❒ What types of drug interactions can occur with the oral contraceptives?

Numerous interactions can occur usually resulting from effects on microsomal drug metabolism. They can induce these enzymes or inhibit them or their effects can be altered by other drugs, which induce enzymes that metabolize the contraceptives. Also some antibiotics kill gut flora involved in enterohepatic recirculation and decrease contraceptive concentration.

❒❒ How do the progestin only minipills work?

They are taken daily, not cyclically. Contraception is due to effects on fertilization and implantation. Ovulation often still occurs so contraception is due to other effects.

❒❒ What is the advantage of these progestin only minipills?

They avoid the adverse effects of the estrogens.

❒❒ How are the progestins only mini pills used?

They are used where estrogens are contraindicated and some pregnancy risk is tolerable, such as in breast-feeding, breast cancer, migraine, hypertension, and older smokers.

❒❒ What long acting progesterone preparations are available?

IUDs with slow-release progesterone, depoprovera (IM injections of medroxyprogesterone acetate every three months), and norplant (levonorgestrel implants).

❒❒ What are the levonorgestrel implants?

Surgical implants of 6 slow release tubes placed under the skin. The effects last 5-6 years and fertility returns following removal of these tubes.

❒❒ What is the rationale for a post-coital contraceptive?

Estrogen alone or estrogen plus progestin taken in high doses for several days within a few days of intercourse can prevent pregnancy.

❒❒ What is the mechanism of action of the post-coital contraceptives?

They may inhibit or delay ovulation, inhibit fertilization and/or implantation. Withdrawal leads to menstruation.

❏❏ **What is the emergency contraceptive kit that is now available?**

Four tablets with moderately high doses of ethinyl estradiol plus levonorgestrel plus a pregnancy test to rule out pre-existing pregnancy. Two pills are taken within 72 hours of intercourse and 2 more 12 hours later.

❏❏ **What is the emergency contraceptive kit used for?**

It is not for routine use as morning after pills, but for rape, incest and medical necessity.

❏❏ **Name some of the agents available for inducing ovulation.**

Bromocriptine, danazol, clomiphene, human chorionic gonadotropin, menotropins, urofollitropin and gonadorelin.

❏❏ **What is human chorionic gonadotropin (hCG)?**

A peptide with activity very similar to LH but with a longer duration of action. It is derived from the urine of pregnant women and given IM.

❏❏ **What is hCG used for?**

It is used to induce ovulation and to treat male infertility. It is also used to treat hypogonadism in both sexes.

❏❏ **What is clomiphene?**

An orally effective anti-estrogen.

❏❏ **What is the mechanism of action of clomiphene?**

It inhibits estrogen feedback on gonadotropin release. The increase in gonadotropins stimulates the ovaries.

❏❏ **How is clomiphene used?**

It induces ovulation in 80% of women and pregnancy in half of those. It is also effective for oligospermia in males.

❏❏ **How is bromocriptine used?**

In cases of infertility due to excess secretion of prolactin.

❏❏ **What is the mechanism of action of bromocriptine?**

It is a dopamine agonist and it inhibits prolactin secretion by activating pituitary dopamine receptors.

❒❒ What is danazol?

Another anti-estrogen.

❒❒ When is danazol used clinically?

It is used if the problem is due to endometriosis. It relieves endometriosis and may increase fertility.

❒❒ What are the menotropins?

Human menopausal gonadotropins. They are derived from the urine of postmenopausal women. They are not orally effective.

❒❒ What is the mechanism of action of the menotropins?

They have both LH and FSH activity.

❒❒ How are the menotropins used?

They are used together with hCG to induce ovulation. Low doses of menotropins plus hCG for 9-12 days are necessary for follicular development. Then large doses of hCG alone are given to simulate the LH surge and induce ovulation. They are also used in preparation for in vitro fertilization. The combination also promotes spermatogenesis in men.

❒❒ What is gonadorelin?

Synthetic gonadotropin releasing hormone (GnRH).

❒❒ How is gonadorelin used clinically?

It is given by pulsatile administration and is used to induce ovulation if the hypothalamus is defective.

❒❒ What are androgens?

Androgens are a group of 19-carbon steroids derived from cholesterol.

❒❒ Where is testosterone produced and how is its secretion regulated?

It is secreted from the testes under control of gonadotropins from anterior pituitary which are under control of GnRH from hypothalamus. Females secrete androgen from ovaries under gonadotropin control. Both males and females secrete androgens from the adrenal gland.

❒❒ What is the physiological role of the androgens?

They are responsible for masculinization during fetal development; for growth spurt and development of make characteristics at puberty; for maintenance of secondary male features throughout life.

❑❑ What androgenic/anabolic steroids are available?

Testosterone (parenteral and scrotal patch), various testosterone esters (for IM injection), Methyltestosterone and fluoxymesterone (orally effective). Oxandrolone and oxymetholone and many others designed to provide anabolic effects with less masculinizing side effects.

❑❑ What are the therapeutic uses of the androgens?

Their major use is in replacement therapy for androgenic effects in prepuberal or postpuberal hypogonadism, hypopituitarism; to induce or maintain secondary sexual characteristics and to prevent osteoporosis in male hypogonadism. They are also used for anabolic effects in tissue wasting; limited use in breast cancer and for the promotion of erythropoiesis in some forms of anemia.

❑❑ What are the adverse effects of the androgens?

Masculinization in women and prepuberal boys (hirsutism, deep voice, clitoral enlargement, decreased breast size and baldness. Feminization can occur in men, due to conversion of androgens to estrogens. Testicular atrophy, oligospermia (due to inhibition of gonadotropin secretion), prostatic enlargement, stimulation of growth of prostatic cancer; acne; liver disease, tumors; Unfavorable changes in serum lipids (with 17-alkyl synthetics); salt and water retention; hypertension and psychosis and violent behavior.

❑❑ What compounds can act as antiandrogens?

GnRH analogs such as leuprolide and others; flutamide; spironolactone; cyproterone; ketoconazole and finasteride.

❑❑ What is the mechanism by which GnRH analogs act as antiandrogens?

Their continuous administration down regulates gonadotropin release and androgen production.

❑❑ How are the GnRH analogs used clinically?

They are used together with flutamide to treat prostate cancer.

❑❑ What is flutamide?

A non-steroidal androgen receptor antagonist.

❑❑ How is flutamide used clinically?

It is used together with GnRH agonists to treat prostate cancer. Flutamide blocks the receptor effects of testosterone especially early in course of GnRH agonist therapy. It is also used for hirsutism in women.

❑❑ What is spironolactone?

An antagonist at mineralocorticoid and androgen receptors. It also inhibits androgen synthesis.

❑❑ What is spironolactone used for clinically?

It is used alone or with oral contraceptives to treat hirsutism in women.

❑❑ What is finasteride?

A 5α reductase inhibitor. It blocks conversion of testosterone to dihydrotestosterone, thus blocking the subset of testosterone effects mediated by dihydrotestosterone.

❑❑ How is finasteride used clinically?

It is used to treat benign prostatic hypertrophy.

❑❑ What is retinoic acid?

All trans-retinoic acid or tretinoin is the acid form of vitamin A.

❑❑ What is tretinoin used for clinically?

It is used for the topical treatment of acne vulgaris.

❑❑ What are the most common adverse effects of topical retinoic acid?

Erythema and dryness occur within the first few weeks of use.

❑❑ What is the mechanism of action of retinoid acid?

Retinoic acid influences gene expression by combining with nuclear receptors. Multiple retinoic acid receptors have been described. They belong to a receptor superfamily that includes receptors for steroids and thyroid hormones and calcitriol.

❑❑ What is isotretinoin?

A synthetic retinoid currently restricted to the treatment of severe cystic acne that is recalcitrant to standard therapies.

❑❑ How does isotretinoin work in the treatment of acne?

The precise mechanism of action is not known although it appears to act by inhibiting sebaceous gland size and function.

❑❑ What are the common adverse effects associated with the use of isotretinoin?

The effects resemble hypervitaminosis A and include dryness and itching of the skin and mucus membranes.

❑❑ What is a major risk for patients taking isotretinoin?

Teratogenicity, therefore women of childbearing potential must use an effective form of contraception for at least 1 month before, throughout therapy and for one or more menstrual cycles following discontinuance of treatment.

❑❑ What effects do the prostaglandins have on uterine motility?

Prostaglandins E_2, E_1 and $F_{2\alpha}$ stimulate uterine contractions. The sensitivity increases as pregnancy progresses. Prostaglandins also induce cervical ripening at low concentrations that do not alter uterine motility. They stimulate GI smooth muscle and can cause vomiting and diarrhea and they also constrict vascular smooth muscle.

❑❑ What forms of prostaglandins are available clinically?

Dinoprostone (PGE_2); carboprost (15-methyl $PGF_{2\,\alpha}$) and misoprostol (PGE_1).

❑❑ What are the therapeutic uses of the prostaglandins as a result of their effects on the uterus?

The major use is in second trimester abortions. Local application of dinoprostone is effective for cervical ripening.

❑❑ What are the ergot alkaloids?

Plant compounds that increase frequency and force of uterine contractions. They also constrict vascular smooth muscle.

❑❑ Which ergot alkaloids are used clinically?

Ergonovine and methylergonovine.

❑❑ What are the therapeutic uses of the ergot alkaloids?

They are primarily used post-partum or following abortion to control bleeding and to induce and maintain uterine contraction.

❑❑ What is meant by the term tocolytic?

It refers to drugs that inhibit uterine motility.

❑❑ How are tocolytics used clinically?

They are used to delay or prevent delivery or to delay or stop labor for brief periods to facilitate other therapeutic measures.

❑❑ What agents are used as tocolytics?

α_2 – adrenergic receptor agonists and magnesium salts.

❑❑ Which α_2 agonist is most commonly used as a tocolytic?

Ritodrine.

❒❒ How is ritodrine used clinically?

It is given IV to stop labor and then switched to oral administration for maintenance.

❒❒ How are magnesium salts used clinically?

Magnesium sulfate is given IV to control eclamptic seizures and to inhibit uterine motility. Magnesium gluconate given orally may be useful for maintenance of tocolysis. Tocolysis is attained at concentrations that do not inhibit cardiac and neuromuscular conduction. High concentrations can lead to respiratory depression and cardiac arrest.

GASTROINTESTINAL PHARMACOLOGY

❑❑ **What are the neural pathways involved in GI motility and secretion?**

CNS (sympathetic and parasympathetic) and the myenteric nervous system.

❑❑ **What other pathways are involved in motility and secretion of the GI tract?**

Hormonal and immunological.

❑❑ **What are the causes of diarrhea?**

Infection, malabsorption, allergy/inflammation, drugs, and hormone secreting tumors.

❑❑ **What non-drug approaches to antidiarrheal therapy are there?**

Patience, rehydration fluids and proper diet and possibly adjustment of dosage or change in medication.

❑❑ **When are antibiotics used for therapy of diarrhea?**

When a specific infectious agent is identified as the cause.

❑❑ **What drugs are the mainstays of nonspecific antidiarrheal therapy?**

Opioid agonists.

❑❑ **Why are codeine and paregoric usually not used?**

They are effective but have a high abuse potential.

❑❑ **What opioids are usually used?**

Diphenoxylate and loperamide.

❑❑ **What are the advantages of these over other opioids?**

They penetrate poorly into the CNS and produce antidiarrheal effects at doses that produce few central effects.

❑❑ **What is the purpose of the atropine that is usually added to the diphenoxylate?**

It discourages abuse because it has unpleasant side effects at high doses.

❒❒ What accounts for the antidiarrheal action of bismuth salts?

Bismuth has antisecretory and antibacterial properties.

❒❒ What are the adverse effects of bismuth salts?

Black staining of the oral cavity and stools and tinnitus.

❒❒ What is the rationale for using octreotide in the treatment of diarrhea?

Octreotide is a peptide analog of somatostatin, a hormone with antisecretory activity. Octreotide mimics its actions but it is more potent and longer lasting.

❒❒ When is octreotide used?

It is used for some hypersecretory tumors and AIDS related diarrhea.

❒❒ What adverse effects does octreotide have?

Nausea and gastrointestinal upset.

❒❒ Describe the pathophysiology of constipation?

Constipation is typically due to a combination of decreased intestinal and colonic motility and excessive fluid uptake. It is not a disease but a symptom that may result from a broad variety of underlying causes.

❒❒ What are some of the causes of constipation?

Congenital, inadequate dietary fiber and fluid ingestion, ignoring the defecatory urge, various drugs and toxins, various neurogenic, metabolic and endocrine conditions and certain structural abnormalities in the GI tract.

❒❒ What is the aim of anti-constipation therapy?

To increase the water content and to encourage intestinal motility.

❒❒ What non-drug approaches are available for the treatment of constipation?

Increasing dietary fiber, fluid ingestion, exercise and enemas are used before certain surgical procedures.

❒❒ What are laxatives?

They are drugs that promote the passage of stools.

❒❒ What are the four classes of laxative drugs?

Bulk forming laxatives, saline and osmotic laxatives, stimulant laxatives and stool softeners.

❑❑ What is the mechanism of action of the bulk-forming laxatives?

They absorb large amounts of water and sometimes form gels. They increase fecal mass and stimulate colonic stretch receptors. They also promote fluid retention in the feces.

❑❑ Which agents are considered bulk forming laxatives?

They are natural or semisynthetic polysaccharides and cellulose derivatives. They include agents such as psyllium, methylcellulose, and calcium polycarbophil.

❑❑ What are some of the adverse effects of drugs in this class?

They have few side effects with few systemic effects. Allergic reactions may occur especially with the plant gums. Flatulence occurs occasionally. Patients should take these with a glass of water otherwise intestinal obstruction and impaction may occur.

❑❑ What is the mechanism of action of the osmotic laxatives?

They are poorly and slowly absorbed and act by their osmotic properties to increase fluid retention in stools and increase the lumen fluid contents.

❑❑ Name two saline laxatives?

Magnesium hydroxide and magnesium sulfate.

❑❑ What is the mechanism of action of the saline laxatives?

They are poorly absorbed ions that favor osmotic movement of water into the lumen.

❑❑ What adverse effects are associated with the use of the saline laxatives?

Excessive laxation, in addition there is a danger of up to 20% of the salts being absorbed and thus they must be avoided in congestive heart failure, renal impairment and the elderly.

❑❑ Name three osmotic laxatives?

Mannitol, lactulose and sorbitol.

❑❑ What is the mechanism of action of the stimulant laxatives?

They promote accumulation of water and electrolytes and stimulate peristalsis. They work by several complex mechanisms on the gut.

❑❑ What are some of the adverse effects for the stimulant laxatives?

The major dangers are fluid and electrolyte deficits resulting from excessive laxative effects. There may be acute effects like cramping and vomiting and long-term effects like electrolyte disturbances, fat malabsorption, fat-soluble vitamin deficiency and laxative dependence.

❒❒ Name three stimulant laxatives?

Bisacodyl, senna and castor oil.

❒❒ How do the stool softeners work?

They act primarily as stool-wetting and stool-softening agents allowing the mixing of water, lipids and other fecal material.

❒❒ Name two stool softeners?

Mineral oil and sodium docusate.

❒❒ What is a major difference between mineral oil and docusate?

Mineral oil can inhibit the absorption of fat-soluble vitamins.

❒❒ What are the potential toxicities of this group?

Generally they have mild side effects but there is the potential for an increase in intestinal absorption and toxicity of other drugs given concurrently.

❒❒ What is meant by laxative abuse?

Laxative abuse occurs during the repeated use of laxatives, which can lead to laxative dependent constipation, chronic diarrhea and electrolyte disturbances.

❒❒ Which groups of laxatives are most commonly abused?

The stimulant laxatives.

❒❒ How do you treat laxative abuse?

Discontinue all laxative use, emphasize the use of dietary fiber by the patient, and make sure the patient has adequate fluid intake and regular physical activity.

❒❒ What are the dangers of laxative abuse?

It may lead to serious GI disturbances, such as the irritable bowel syndrome.

❒❒ What is inflammatory bowel disease?

A set of conditions characterized by inflammation of the colon and or intestinal lining. The condition is chronic with temporary remissions. There are familial and infectious components to it.

❒❒ What are the symptoms of inflammatory bowel disease?

Diarrhea, pain, bleeding and related deficiencies.

❑❑ What are the two major types of inflammatory bowel disease?

Ulcerative colitis and Crohn's disease.

❑❑ What is the difference between ulcerative colitis and Crohn's disease

Crohn's disease is more extensive in nature as it extends to the small intestine and deeper into the intestinal walls.

❑❑ What are the four groups of drugs that are used to treat inflammatory bowel disease?

Corticosteroids, 5-aminosalicylic acid derivatives, infliximab and immunosuppressives.

❑❑ What are the two aminosalicylic acid derivatives used to treat inflammatory bowel disease?

Mesalamine and sulfasalazine.

❑❑ What is the mechanism of action of the salicylic acid derivatives?

They inhibit prostaglandin and leukotriene synthesis.

❑❑ How are they used clinically?

They are used for mild to moderately active disease.

❑❑ How do sulfasalazine and mesalamine differ from each other?

Sulfasalazine combines suflapyridine plus 5-aminosalicylic acid while mesalamine is just 5-aminosalicylic acid. The sulfapyridine functions mainly to deliver mesalamine to the colon but accounts for most of its side effects.

❑❑ What is infliximab?

A monoclonal antibody that binds tumor necrosis factor.

❑❑ How is infliximab used clinically?

It is given by I.V. injection for the treatment of inflammatory bowel disease.

❑❑ What immunosuppressive agents are used in treating inflammatory bowel disease?

Azathioprine, methotrexate and cyclosporine as well as a few others.

❑❑ How are the immunosuppressives used clinically in inflammatory bowel disease?

They have steroid sparing properties. They are usually used in more serious disease.

❒❒ What area of the body coordinates the emetic response?

The vomiting center in the brain.

❒❒ What areas input into the vomiting center to mediate vomiting?

There are many inputs including the chemoreceptor trigger zone (CTZ), the vestibular apparatus, the higher brainstem and cortical structures, visceral afferents in the periphery, and emetic substances in the circulation.

❒❒ What receptors or signalling pathways mediate emesis and nausea?

5-HT_3 receptors, dopamine D2 receptors, H_1 histamine receptors, and cholinergic receptors.

❒❒ What are the major groups of antiemetic agents?

D2 antagonists, 5-HT_3 antagonists, corticosteroids and cannabinoids, antihistamines, muscarinic antagonists and the benzodiazepines.

❒❒ What are the advantages of combination antiemetic therapy?

It can result in a major improvement in the ability to reduce nausea and vomiting and a decrease in toxicity.

❒❒ How are the HT_3 antagonists like ondansetron used clinically?

To prevent and minimize emesis due to moderate-high doses of chemotherapy e.g. cisplatin and radiation.

❒❒ How are the HT_3 antagonists administered?

Orally or IV as a single dose.

❒❒ What are the adverse effects of the 5-HT_3 antagonists?

They have transient, mild adverse effects, including headache, GI effects, lightheadedness and sedation.

❒❒ What is the big advantage of using the 5-HT_3 antagonists as antiemetics?

They lack the extrapyramidal side effects associated with metoclopramide.

❒❒ What is the mechanism of action of metoclopramide as an antiemetic?

It is a D2 dopamine receptor antagonist.

❒❒ Name three other groups of D2 dopamine receptor antagonist antiemetics besides metoclopramide?

Phenothiazines, benzimidazoles such as domperidone and butyrophenones (e.g. haloperidol).

❑❑ What are the adverse effects associated with use of metoclopramide?

Antidopaminergic effects including extrapyramidal reactions, anxiety and depression.

❑❑ How are the corticosteroids used as antiemetics?

They are used in combination with other therapies to enhance overall antiemetic effects and to reduce the severity and incidence of some adverse effects.

❑❑ What are the adverse effects associated with the use of the cannabinoids as antiemetics?

Hallucinations, disorientation and vertigo.

❑❑ What type of neural regulation is involved in gastric motility?

Stimulation by cholinergic neurons, inhibition by adrenergic neurons and a modulatory influence by the enteric nervous system in which dopamine and serotonin play a role.

❑❑ What drugs can be used to treat gastric hypomotility?

Antiemetic phenothiazines, bethanechol and prokinetic agents.

❑❑ What are the major prokinetic drugs?

Metoclopramide, cisapride and domperidone.

❑❑ How does cisapride work?

It increases colonic motility and can cause diarrhea. It is devoid of dopamine antagonist activity.

❑❑ What are the therapeutic uses of cisapride?

Disorders of gastric hypomotility, gastroesophogeal reflux disease, gastroparetic conditions and chronic idiopathic constipation and colonic hypomotility.

❑❑ What are the adverse effects of cisapride?

Arrhythmias. Transient abdominal cramping and diarrhea. It may also increase the absorption of diazepam and alcohol.

❑❑ What are the pathways regulating gastric acid secretion?

Neural stimulation via the vagus nerve, endocrine stimulation via gastrin released from antral G cells, and paracrine stimulation by local release of histamine from enterochromaffin-like cells.

❑❑ **What signalling pathways are involved in gastric acid production?**

cAMP mediated pathways (H_2 receptors) and calcium mediated pathways (gastrin and acetylcholine).

❑❑ **What is the final common pathway in acid production by all three mediators?**

Activation of the H^+/K^+ ATPase proton pump.

❑❑ **What are the mechanisms of protective adaptation in the parietal cells?**

Prostaglandin production and production of mucus and bicarbonate.

❑❑ **What are the causes of peptic ulcer?**

H.pylori infection, treatment with non steroidal antiinflammatory drugs (NSAIDS), and hypersecretory tumors.

❑❑ **How is *H.pylori* infection diagnosed?**

Mainly by measurement of isotopic ammonia released by the urease production.

❑❑ **How does *H.pylori* infection cause ulcers?**

Through release of ammonia from urease production by the bacteria and through cytokines produced in reaction to the inflammation produced by the bacteria.

❑❑ **What are the different targets for treatment of peptic ulcer?**

Neutralize the gastric acid, prevent acid secretion. enhance cytoprotection and eliminate *H.pylori* infection.

❑❑ **What is the mechanism of action of the antacids used to treat peptic ulcer?**

They are weak bases that directly neutralize stomach acid.

❑❑ **Name some of the commonly used antacids?**

Magnesium and aluminum hydroxides, sodium bicarbonate or calcium salts.

❑❑ **How are the antacids used clinically?**

They are effective in promoting healing of duodenal ulcers, but their benefit in gastric ulcers is less clear. They are also used for quick relief of heartburn but other drugs are preferred.

❑❑ **What are the adverse effects associated with use of the antacids?**

Compliance problems due to their unpleasant taste, ingestion volumes and dosing schedule. There might be a change in bowel habits since magnesium salts often have a cathartic effect and aluminum hydroxide may be constipating. There may also be problems related to cation absorption and systemic alkalosis.

❑❑ What types of drug-drug interactions are associated with the antacids?

They may alter the rates of dissolution, absorption, bioavailability and elimination of a number of drugs.

❑❑ How do the H_2 receptor antagonists work?

They are histamine congeners that contain a bulky side chain in place of the ethylamine moiety. They block acid secretion from parietal cells that is stimulated by histamine. They can reduce acid production by as much as 90%.

❑❑ What are the clinical uses of the H_2 receptor antagonists?

They are used for the healing and prevention of duodenal and gastic ulcers, for the Zollinger-Ellison syndrome and for treating esophageal reflux and dyspepsia.

❑❑ Name the four major histamine H_2 receptor antagonists?

Cimetidine, ranitidine, famotidine and nizatidine.

❑❑ What are the adverse effects of cimetidine?

Production of a confusional state, reversible gynecomastia, elevation in serum prolactin and alteration in estrogen metabolism. It can also inhibit drug metabolizing enzymes so their may be many potential drug-drug interactions.

❑❑ How do the adverse effects of the other antagonists differ from cimetidine?

They lack the antiandrogenic actions associated with cimetidine. They have no effects on cytochrome P450 enzymes unlike cimetidine and headache occurs in 34% of people taking famotidine or ranitidine.

❑❑ What is the mechanism of action of the proton pump inhibitors?

They irreversible block the H^+/K^+ ATPase pump. They are prodrugs requiring activation in the local acidic environment.

❑❑ How are they used therapeutically?

For short-term treatment of gastric and duodenal ulcers and for esophageal reflux and hypersecretory conditions.

❑❑ What are the adverse effects of the proton pump inhibitors?

They are well tolerated with some GI upset. There is concern about their long term use and possible increase in cancer. They also inhibit cytochrome P450 enzymes and may interact with drugs metabolized by that system.

❒❒ What proton pump inhibitors are clinically available?

Omeprazole, lansoprazole and raberprazole.

❒❒ What is misoprostol?

A prostaglandin E_1 analog.

❒❒ What is the mechanism of action of misoprostol?

It down regulates acid secretion from parietal cells.

❒❒ How is misoprostol used clinically?

It is useful prophylactically for patients on extended NSAID therapy. It prevents gastric and duodenal ulcers in these patients.

❒❒ What are the adverse effects of misoprostol?

A dose dependent diarrhea is most common. Also some nausea is produced and there may be unwanted uterine contractions.

❒❒ What is sucralfate?

A mucosal protective agent.

❒❒ What is the mechanism of action of sucralfate?

It is an aluminum sucrose sulfate that gels at pH <4. It selectively binds to necrotic tissue protecting the ulcer site from acid and pepsin insults.

❒❒ What are the clinical uses of sucralfate?

To promote healing of ulcers.

❒❒ Does sucralfate produce any adverse effects?

Constipation and dry mouth can occur and it also binds some drugs reducing their bioavailability.

❒❒ Can sulcralfate be taken with the proton pump inhibitors and the H_2 receptor blockers?

No, because sucralfate requires an acid pH to be activated and thus should not be given simultaneously with drugs of either class as they reduce acid production.

❒❒ What mechanism accounts for the anti-ulcer effects of bismuth salts?

Selective binding to ulcer craters, inhibition of pepsin activity and stimulation of mucus secretion. Its greatest benefit is probably from its antibacterial action toward *H.pylori*.

❑❑ What is the preferred treatment for patients with peptic ulcers who test positive for *H.pylori*?

Combination therapy with an acid blocker or pump inhibitor plus antibiotics.

❑❑ What is the rationale behind this combined treatment?

Acid blockers promote healing but don't prevent recurrences. Antibiotics prevent recurrences by eliminating the causative bacteria but don't promote healing.

❑❑ Why should combinations of antibiotics be used instead of just one?

To avoid resistance.

❑❑ Which antibiotic with activity vs. *H.pylori* is associated with the most incidences of resistance?

Metronidazole.

❑❑ Which antibiotic-acid blocker combination has provided the best results?

Clarithromycin plus amoxicillin plus lansoprazole for 14 days.

RENAL PHARMACOLOGY

❒❒ What are diuretics?

They are drugs that are used to increase the rate of urine flow.

❒❒ What is the main mechanism of action of diutetics?

They affect ion transport in the nephron. The clinically useful ones primarily inhibit sodium reabsorption with water being carried along passively.

❒❒ What are the general uses for the diuretics?

They are the cornerstones for the treatment of edema or volume overload, particularly that due to congestive heart failure, ascites, chronic renal failure and nephrotic syndrome.

❒❒ What non-edematous conditions are the diuretics used for?

Nephrolithiasis/hypercalcuria, hypercalcemia, diabetes insipidus, hypertension, glaucoma and cerebral edema.

❒❒ What are the major groups of diuretics?

Carbonic anhydrase inhibitors, loop diuretics, thiazide diuretics, osmotic diuretics and the potassium sparing diuretics.

❒❒ What osmotic diuretics are commonly used?

Mannitol, urea and isosorbide.

❒❒ What is the mechanism of action of the osmotic diuretics?

They are freely filterable substances that are not reabsorbed in the nephron. The presence of a non-reabsorbable solution in the nephron reduces water reabsorption through an osmotic effect, thereby impairing the ability of the proximal tubule and thick ascending limb to reabsorb sodium.

❒❒ How is mannitol used clinically?

Because of the availability of the loop diuretics the osmotic diuretics are used mainly for nondiuretic uses. Mannitol is highly effective in treating cerebral edema and is used frequently in neurosurgical procedures, in head trauma and in patients with fulminant hepatic failure awaiting transplants who develop increased intracranial pressure. It is also used for the reduction of intraocular pressure prior to eye surgery and mannitol has been used in patients with acute renal failure in attempts to “open up” the kidney.

❒❒ What adverse effects are associated with the use of the osmotic diuretics?

Expansion of the extracellular fluid volume, which could be detrimental to the heart. Excessive use of mannitol without adequate water replacement can ultimately lead to severe dehydration, free water loss and hypernatremia.

❒❒ What reaction is catalyzed by carbonic anhydrase?

$CO_2 + H_2O \rightarrow H_2CO_3 \rightarrow H^+ + HCO_3^-$

❒❒ How efficient are the carbonic anhydrase inhibitors as diuretics?

They are only weak diuretics because other sites along the nephron compensate for the effects of the carbonic anhydrase inhibitors.

❒❒ What is the prototypical carbonic anhydrase inhibitor?

Acetazolamide.

❒❒ What is the mechanism of action of the carbonic anhydrase inhibitors?

They inhibit carbonic anhydrase. The H^+ produced by the breakdown of carbonic acid is usually exchanged for Na^+ and is also used to combine with bicarbonate in the lumen. Without the H^+, there is decreased reabsorption of Na^+ and bicarbonate, which results in diuresis.

❒❒ What are the therapeutic uses of the carbonic anhydrase inhibitors?

They are used infrequently as diuretics. They are used for treatment of edema due to congestive heart failure and for some drug-induced edemas. However, the major indication is open-angle glaucoma. Acetazolamide is also used for the treatment of epilepsy and it also provides symptomatic relief in patients with acute mountain sickness. These drugs are also used to correct metabolic alkalosis.

❒❒ What are the adverse effects of the carbonic anhydrase inhibitors?

Metabolic acidosis and potassium depletion are the primary adverse effects of these drugs. Some of the adverse effects are similar to that of the sulfonamides including fever, formation of urinary calculi, crystalluria and exfoliative dermatitis.

❒❒ Name some thiazide diuretics?

Chlorothiazide, hydrochlorothiazide, metolazone and indapamide.

❒❒ How do the thiazide diuretics work?

They act at the distal convoluted tubule to block coupled NaCl transport. They bind to the chloride binding site of the NaCl transporter.

❒❒ How do the thiazides effect electrolyte excretion?

There is increased excretion of Na^+, Cl^-, K^+ and H_2O, but decreased calcium excretion. While the loop diuretics inhibit Ca^{++} reabsorption, thiazides actually enhance calcium reabsorption in the distal convoluted tubule.

❑❑ **How effective are the thiazides as diuretics?**

They are only moderately effective since approximately 90% of the filtered load is reabsorbed before reaching the distal convoluted tubule.

❑❑ **What are the thiazide diuretics used for?**

Their greatest use has been in the treatment of hypertension. They are also used to treat edema, nephrogenic diabetes insipidus and hypercalcuria.

❑❑ **What are the major distinguishing features among the different thiazides?**

Cost and duration of action.

❑❑ **What adverse effects are produced after the thiazides are used?**

Alterations in plasma K^+ (hypokalemia), elevation of plasma urate, hyperlipidemia, hyperglycemia and hypersensitivity reactions (the thiazides are sulfonamides).

❑❑ **Name three loop diuretics?**

Furosemide, bumetanide and ethacrynic acid.

❑❑ **What is another name for the loop diuretics?**

High ceiling diuretics. The name comes from the fact that they have the highest efficacy of all groups of diuretics.

❑❑ **What is the reason for this high efficacy of the loop diuretics?**

First of all, about 25% of the filtered load is normally reabsorbed by the thick ascending limb and secondly nephron segments past the thick limb do not possess the reabsorptive capacity to fully compensate.

❑❑ **What is the mechanism of action of the loop diuretics?**

They act at the ascending limb of the loop of Henle to block Na^+ reabsorption. They bind to and inhibit the Na^+-K^+ $2Cl^-$ transporter in the thick ascending limb of the loop of Henle.

❑❑ **What is the renal response to these drugs?**

Increased excretion of Na^+, Cl^-, K^+ and water.

❑❑ **Which of the loop diuretics is a prodrug?**

Ethacrynic acid is metabolized; the cysteine conjugate is the active form while furosemide and bumetanide act as parent compounds.

❏❏ How are the loop diuretics used clinically?

They are used to treat edema. They should be reserved for situations where very efficacious diuretics are needed. Loop diuretics are the most effective diuretics available. Many patients, particularly those with severe heart failure, severe cirrhosis, nephrotic syndrome and renal insufficiency require loop diuretics rather than less efficacious diuretics. A major use is in acute pulmonary edema.

❏❏ What are the major adverse effects associated with the use of the loop diuretics?

Fluid and electrolyte imbalances (hyponatremia and hypokalemia) as well as ototoxicity that are seen as tinnitus, hearing impairment, deafness, vertigo and a sense of fullness in the ears.

❏❏ What are the potassium sparing diuretics?

Spironolactone, amiloride and triamterene.

❏❏ What the term potassium sparing diuretic means?

Diuretics that produce little or no increase in K^+ excretion.

❏❏ Describe the mechanism of action of the potassium sparing diuretics?

They primarily inhibit the passage of sodium in the luminal fluid into the principal cells of the late distal convoluted tubule and cortical collecting tubule. This then prevents the movement of potassium from these cells into the luminal fluid.

❏❏ How does spironolactone work?

It is an aldosterone antagonist.

❏❏ How does triamterene work?

It is an inhibitor of renal epithelial sodium channels. It blocks sodium reabsorption that facilitates K^+ entry into the nephron.

❏❏ What is the renal response to the potassium sparing diuretics?

There is a modest increase in the excretion of Na^+, chloride and water.

❏❏ How is spironolactone used clinically?

It is used to treat primary hyperaldosteronism and edematous states caused by secondary aldosteronism especially cirrhosis, nephrotic syndrome and cardiac failure.

❑❑ What adverse effects are associated with the use of spironolactone?

Gynecomastia and impotence as a result of the similarity of spironolactone to progesterone.

❑❑ How are the nonsteroidal potassium sparing diuretics used clinically?

In edematous states, usually in combination with other diuretics, particularly thiazides.

❑❑ What are the adverse effects of the potassium sparing diuretics?

The most dangerous effect is hyperkalemia. Triampterene also can reduce glucose tolerance and induce photosensitization and has been associated with interstitial nephritis and renal stones. Metabolic acidosis also may occur

❑❑ What electrolyte change characterizes almost all diuretics?

A loss of potassium ions.

❑❑ Which diuretic produces a reduction in insulin release from the pancreas?

Chlorothiazide and other thiazides.

❑❑ Which diuretics enhance the parathyroid hormone-mediated reabsorption of calcium in the distal tubule?

Hydrochlorothiazide and other thiazides.

BIBLIOGRAPHY

Antimicrobial Therapy and Vaccines. edited by V.L.Yu, T.C.Merigan, and S.L. Barriere Baltimore, Williams and Wilkins, 1999.

Basic and Clinical Pharmacology 7th Ed. B.G. Katzung. Stamford, Conn., Appleton and Lange, 1998.

Brater, D.C. Pharmacology of Diuretics Am J. Med. Sci. *319*: 38 (2000)

Bylund, D., Berndt, W., Hexum, T., Deupree, J., Murrin, C., Scholar, E., Monaghan, D., Toews, M and Kawahara, R., *Syllabus for the Medical, Pharmacy and Graduate Pharmacology Course*, Univ. Nebraska College of Medicine, 1999-2000.

Claesson, H.-E. And Dahlen, S.-E. J.Internal Med. Asthma and leukotrienes: antileukotrienes as novel antiasthmatic drugs.245: 205 (1999)

Drugs for Asthma.The Medical Letter 42:19 (2000).

Goodman and Gilman's, *The pharmacological basis of therapeutics.* 9th Ed. edited by J.G., Hardman, L.E. Limbird, P.B. Molinoff, R.W. Ruddon and A.G. Gilman. New York: Mc Graw-Hill, 1996.

Graham,D.Y. *Therapy of Helicobacter pylori*: Current Status and Issues. Gastroenterology *118*:S2-S8, 2000.

Heart Disease. A textbook of Cardiovascular Medicine. 5th Ed. edited by E.Braunwald. Philadelphia. W.B. Saunders,

Hollister, L. and Claghorn, J., New Antidepressants. Ann. Rev. Pharmacol. Toxicol. 32: 165 (1993).

Pharmacology. Brenner, G.M. Philadelphia, W.B. Saunders, 2000

Pharmacology. H.P.Rang, M.M. Dale and J.M. Ritter.4th.ed. New York, Harcourt Brace and Company, 1999.

The Antimicrobial Drugs. 2nd Ed., E.M. Scholar and W.B. Pratt New York, Oxford University Press , 2000

*The Anticancer Drugs.*2nd Ed. W.B Pratt, R.W. Ruddon, W.D Ensminger, and J.Maybaum.. New York, Oxford University Press, 1994

USPDI. Drug Information for the Health Care Professional. Micromedex Inc., 1999.